When Psychological Problems
Mask Medical Disorders

When Psychological Problems Mask Medical Disorders

A Guide for Psychotherapists

JAMES MORRISON

The Guilford Press
New York London

© 1997 The Guilford Press
A Division of Guilford Publications, Inc.
72 Spring Street, New York, NY 10012

Printed in the United States of America

This book is printed on acid-free paper.

Last digit is print number: 9   8   7   6   5   4   3   2   1

Library of Congress Cataloging-in-Publication Data
Morrison, James R., 1940–
    When psychological problems mask medical disorders : a guide
for psychotherapists / James Morrison.
        p.   cm.
    Includes bibliographical references and index.
    ISBN 1-57230-180-5 (hard)
    1. Psychological manifestations of general diseases.   2. Medicine,
Psychosomatic.   I. Title.
    [DNLM: 1. Mental Disorders—diagnosis. 2. Mental Disorders—
etiology. 3. Affective Symptoms—diagnosis. 4. Disease—psychology.
5. Diagnosis, Differential.   WM 141 M879w 1997]
RC455.4.B5M67   1997
616'.01'9—dc21
DNLM/DLC
for Library of Congress   97-17253
                                                                CIP

*This book is dedicated
to Molly Mullikin,
a wonderful secretary
and my good friend*

CONTENTS

INTRODUCTION

Almost always, physical illness has some kind of emotional impact. It stands to reason that having a serious illness will cause anxiety or depression. Yet of the thousands of medical disorders to which humankind is heir, only a few directly cause mental symptoms. This relative handful makes up the subject matter of this book.

The sort of diagnostic problem I have addressed can arise in a variety of contexts:

- One of the most common situations arises when a clinician must determine whether depressive symptoms are caused by a physical disorder, in contrast to a major depressive disorder. An exactly analogous case can be made for symptoms of anxiety or psychosis.
- In another common scenario, the clinician needs to know whether a patient's already-proven physical illness can account for a given set of mental symptoms. Examples might be drawn from the entire contents of this book.
- The diagnosis of somatization disorder and other somatoform disorders has been a staple of mental health differential diagnosis for many years. Unhappily, this is still an area where far too few practitioners, whether in the medical or mental health arenas, have adequate training and experience.
- Over a period of days or weeks, or even longer, you notice a change in your patient's behavior (less reserved, perhaps,

1

or showing mannerisms). Is it caused by the gradual onset of a primary mood disorder or by physical illness?

- Altered appearance, which may be quite external, such as changes in the condition of your patient's skin, or (by inference) internal, as hinted by the beginnings of a limp, a tremor, can herald either physical or mental disease. How does one determine which one? For that matter, how do you even know where to go to find out?

- Your patient is being treated for "typical" symptoms, say, of a depressive disorder but doesn't get well. Could the cause of these symptoms actually be a physical disease?

- Finally, in my experience with somewhere over 15,000 mental health patients, it is distressingly easy—perhaps it is the norm—to see a patient for several months, long enough to become comfortable with the mental health diagnosis for which you are providing treatment. So it is another goal of this book to stimulate practitioners to "think outside the mental health box" and consider other diagnoses for patients with whom they have had long acquaintance.

Each of the above is an instance where knowledge of disease and the diagnostic process can be critical for patients who, if less carefully considered, might continue to be inaccurately diagnosed until incapacitated by a disease that could have been easily corrected if detected earlier.

I don't plan to discuss those conditions (such as uncomplicated asthma) that may be worsened by stress but do not cause mental symptoms themselves. And I have omitted the genitourinary diseases, whose emotional symptoms are primarily sexual—important, of course, but these sexual problems are a bit specialized for most mental health practitioners. Drugs and other toxins have a host of side effects of their own that require entire books to do them justice.

Definitions

I have tried to define the more specialized medical terms I've used and have in most cases redefined them for each section of the book. I apologize for any omissions in this regard.

My usage of several terms deserves some explanation. I have been a bit cavalier with *symptom*. Strictly speaking, a symptom is what the patient complains of (back pain, swollen joints, an anxiety attack, hearing voices), whereas a *sign* is what an observer notices about the patient (reddened skin, swollen joints, worried facial expression, clenched fists). In this book I have allowed symptom to refer to either—it seems perfectly understandable and a bit more relaxed. Until late in the 19th century, the two terms were used more or less interchangeably. Even today, the distinction is not razor sharp: Note that "swollen joints" appears on both of the lists just given as examples.

The term *syndrome* I have used in the traditional sense; that is, it is a collection of symptoms that commonly occur together. (The word has Greek roots, and it means "running together.") Most patients who have any given syndrome will experience some, but not all, of its symptoms.

In assigning degree of rarity to the illnesses described in Part II, I confess to a certain arbitrariness. But epidemiology has yet to become an exact science, and for many of these diseases the data are sparse, contradictory, or even nonexistent. Often, the numbers must be estimated. Nevertheless, for better or for worse, I have tried to categorize all of these illnesses as follows:

Common. Most adults have at least one friend or acquaintance who has, or will have, the condition in question. The prevalence ranges to as low as 1 in 200.

Frequent. A town or small city will be home to one or more of these people. Frequency ranges downward from 1 in 200 to 1 in 10,000.

Uncommon. There will be at least one such person in a large city (or small state). These patients occur as infrequently as 1 in 500,000. When one is identified, it is often cause for a grand rounds presentation in a hospital or medical school.

Rare. Less frequent than 1 in 1 million. When encountered, such a patient is likely to be written up in a medical journal.

Keep in mind that the frequencies stated are those of the illnesses themselves—mental complications will generally occur in only a minority of cases. Also note that the frequencies are given in terms of lifetime prevalence—the likelihood that a person will develop the illness at some time prior to death.

In discussing evaluation, I have tried to indicate only the one or two tests that are the simplest, most helpful, or most commonly used. Of course, the workup of most patients will include far more tests and procedures than can be usefully described in a book of this nature.

Using This Book

I have designed this book to be used in a number of ways.

1. Use the first portion of Part I as a guide to the sorts of observations you can make that might indicate a physical disorder. I have arranged these within the framework of the typical mental status examination (MSE), familiar to any mental health professional. The descriptions given here will point the way to some of the illnesses discussed later in the book.

2. Part II discusses some 60 disorders that can have important implications for mental health patients. You can learn something about the typical appearance (physical and mental) of patients who have these disorders. Of course, the disorders can include many symptoms besides those I have detailed in this section, which attempts only to list those that are most important, common, or prominent.

3. Part III cross-tabulates every disorder discussed in Part II against all mental and physical symptoms discussed. At a glance, you can see how, for example, typical neurological symptoms of hypo- and hyperparathyroidism compare.

4. You can also use Part III as an index to the disorders in which any given symptom might be found. But heed the warning that, in medicine, almost anything is possible and that any compilation of symptoms can be neither exhaustive nor exclusive.

5. Finally, in the Appendix I have included a brief, annotated list of suggested readings and other resources for further learning.

I hope that by the time you finish this book, you will be:

- More aware of mental symptoms that occur in the course of physical disease.
- More alert to the physical symptoms (and signs!) that could indicate the need for a medical intervention.
- Increasingly curious about illness beyond the usual interests of the mental health practitioner.

In Appreciation

For their help with this project I want to express my appreciation to several people. They include V. Kay Hafner, Andrew Henry, Barbara Nicholson, and Mary Walters, who have helped me realize anew why it is I so appreciate librarians; the anonymous critics who contributed their time and wisdom; and Mary Morrison, for her usual and unusual support and advice. I especially want to thank G. Arul, MD, Arthur Swislocki, MD, and the many mental health professionals whose after-class comments and requests provided much of the inspiration for this book.

Part I

A REVIEW
OF SYMPTOMS

Melissa Block had her therapist worried. She had been completely healthy until 9 months earlier, when at age 42 she had gradually developed anxiety, nausea, and episodic vomiting. She had also begun to complain of depression, and she seemed to worry obsessively about her health and her family. Abdominal pain, weight loss, and mild lethargy led to several medical evaluations. A physical exam and routine lab studies were all normal, so her family doctor referred her out for psychotherapy. At her first appointment she cried and paced nervously around the room, complaining of depression and trouble sleeping at night.

But 2 months of therapy (combined with an antidepressant drug in doses that would be adequate for most people) had yielded no improvement. Melissa's depression continued unabated, and, truthfully, did not seem excessive in light of her continuing abdominal pain. Recent family problems—her husband had confessed to a long-standing affair with the woman who had once been their real estate agent—suggested an emotional component to her difficulty.

But Melissa had never been one to complain much about her health. As a matter of fact, in the past she had shrugged off worse problems than those she had now, notably the combat death of her first husband and the loss of a baby to sudden infant death syndrome. But with no history of manic symptoms, no family history of mood disorder, and little improvement with treatment, of course, her clinician was worried. This illness did not seem at all like a primary mood disorder. Back to her internist went Melissa for more tests.

Another physical exam and more blood tests were normal, but a repeat of an earlier radiological examination finally struck pay dirt. An upper gastrointestinal (GI) series, this time with small bowel follow-through, revealed a slight shrinking of the lining of the small intestine. It was enough to justify an exploratory laparotomy, which revealed a pancreatic cancer that had invaded Melissa's small intestine.

Happily, most of the disorders that can produce mental symptoms are less serious than pancreatic carcinoma (Melissa died only a few months after the diagnosis was made). Although research has yet to determine what percentage of patients have mental symptoms that are caused or exacerbated by physical disease, it seems safe to guess that every mental health practitioner with an active caseload will have such patients. The lifetime prevalence of the medical disorders described in this book is such that most of us will at some time or other contract at least one. (Of course, in most cases they will not produce mental symptoms.)

The Need for Evaluation

If your patient starts convulsing or coughing up blood, you realize at once that something is wrong. But many symptoms of physical illness are far less obvious. If they develop gradually enough, even life-threatening symptoms may not seem serious.

At first, the patient may not even have physical symptoms— early manifestations may be strictly emotional or behavioral. Like Melissa Block's, they may have been previously investigated and discarded as unimportant. To counteract the potential for confusion, you can use several principles to help determine which symptoms, or syndromes, demand attention:

- *New symptoms.* Of course, the ideal time to detect a new disorder is with the patient's first symptom. The trouble is, the first time a symptom occurs, it might be relatively mild and go unnoticed.

- *More symptoms.* This principle seems pretty obvious. A cough may escape your notice; you will pay far more attention to that cough when it is accompanied by chest pain and fever. Similarly, by itself, a complaint of low mood may not mean very much, but combine it with sleeplessness, weight loss, poor concentration, and guilty ruminations, and you have real cause for concern.
- *Symptoms that are worse.* This also seems nearly self-explanatory. You are more concerned about crushing substernal chest pain than mild heartburn, about an outright panic attack than an occasional twinge of anxiety.
- *Symptoms that persist.* Nearly everyone feels depressed at some time or other, but the feeling usually lasts only a few hours, a day or two at most. Such a "depression," even when the person feels it strongly, usually has no clinical importance. But even a low-grade depression, if it continues day after day, can in important ways affect a person's concentration at school or work and interactions with spouse or friends.
- *Alarming symptoms.* Some symptoms automatically suggest serious disease; a dark spot on the skin could be a melanoma; blood-tinged sputum may indicate tuberculosis; suicidal ideas suggest clinical depression. Serious symptoms are red flags that demand immediate investigation.
- *Symptom patterns.* Symptoms that tend to occur together (a *syndrome*) suggest a disorder with a common cause or for which a particular treatment may be effective. For example, one of the syndromes discussed in this book is normal pressure hydrocephalus, whose classical symptom pattern includes dementia, trouble walking, and urinary incontinence.

As the foregoing principles attest, detection of physical or mental disorders depends on how readily you can recognize changes in your patient's appearance, behavior, physical condition, and emotional state. Sometimes this is easy—the changes are so striking that anyone would notice, or someone (patient, relative) makes a point of reporting them to you. But more subtle

TABLE 1. Clues that Suggest a New or Different Diagnosis

New behaviors

Change in emotions

New physical symptoms

Symptoms that don't fit the working diagnosis

Symptoms that don't resolve, despite apparently adequate treatment

changes are harder to spot, and in a first interview, they can escape your attention completely. That is when discussions with relatives, friends, or other people who know your patient well can be especially valuable. Often, their observations can provide information about the patient's behavior that you won't obtain from any other source. (For convenience, I have listed some of these clues to new diagnoses in Table 1.)

Most of the time, mental symptoms are not caused by medical illness. This fact represents something of a problem for clinicians, who may find it hard to keep physical illness in mind when it doesn't turn up very often. Yet mental health patients can and do develop such disorders, which await identification by the clinician whose mind is prepared. This book will help prepare you to spot medical disorders by giving you the *facts* about diseases as well as the *process* of information gathering by observation. The remainder of Part I will be devoted to the details of this process.

Making an Evaluation

There is a robust literature on the subject of evaluating patients, whether in mental health or in general medicine. Of course, a familiarity with many illnesses is required. And that implies knowledge of the myriad symptoms that are found across the spectrum of human disease. But how do clinicians actually use their information to arrive at a working diagnosis?

There is no simple answer to that question, though a variety of answers have been attempted. Over the past several decades, clinicians have attempted to use a variety of mechanical (either on paper or computers) devices for helping with decision making. Most prominent among these are itemized clinical criteria (such as DSM-IV) and decision trees. Neither of these, nor of the other means that have been devised, appear to substitute adequately for the judgment of an experienced clinician.

Part of the problem may be that these methods fail to replicate the process experienced clinicians use to arrive at a diagnosis. Most clinicians, even very fine ones, would be hard-pressed to describe the mental steps they use. And indeed, although this process has not been adequately studied, there does not seem to be the methodical sifting through data sets or the examining of successive decision points that have been used by machines or decision trees.

1. The first thing an experienced clinician does in making a diagnosis is to arrive at a *preliminary formulation*. This usually occurs very quickly in the course of a diagnostic interview—often within the first minute or two—and may be based on a key observation or pattern of symptoms. Of course, any impression so quickly made may be logically insupportable and based on woefully inadequate data, but at least it identifies a general area (in the case of a mental health patient, anxiety disorders, mood disorders, psychosis) that must be further investigated.

2. The clinician next obtains *further data* (see Table 2) that would support or refute the hypothesis but always remains alert to the possibility of alternative diagnoses.

3. Finally, with enough accumulated data, a *final hypothesis* can be selected. Studies have shown that clinicians are more likely to select the correct diagnosis if they have included it in their initial *differential*—the list of diagnoses that they initially

TABLE 2. Sources of Further Data

Previous information from workups and hospital charts

Interviews with family, friends

Reinterview of patient to pick up missing data

Laboratory exams

Imaging studies (X-ray, computerized tomography [CT scan], MRI)

Psychological testing

Passing of time[a]

[a]The passing of time can be a powerful tool for revealing or verifying diagnoses. Its danger, of course, is that by the time the diagnosis has been uncovered, it may be too late for the patient.

judge could, even if ever so unlikely, be responsible for the symptoms.

Sources of Error

Clinicians can get themselves and their patients into difficulties through a variety of errors in the diagnostic process. Some of these are out-and-out mistakes; others represent the too-vigorous application of otherwise praiseworthy principles. Here are only a few of them:

• *Focusing only on what the clinician knows best.* "If your only tool is a hammer, everything looks like a nail" the saying goes. Broad-based knowledge and receptiveness to new observations help ensure accurate diagnosis.

• *Seeking a comfort level.* Some diagnoses are more comfortable to make than others—they are easier to treat or have a better natural outcome.

• *Relying on an intuitive diagnosis.* With experience, a clinician develops a feel for what is correct diagnostically. Often, this intuition is correct. But because it can come a cropper, the gut-level impression should always be backed up with sound, scientific information (see Table 2).

• *Making snap judgments.* These are related to intuitive diagnoses; both the argument and remedy are the same.

• *Relying on statistics.* If disease "X" is common in the population at hand, clinicians increase their suspicion of "X" in an individual patient. This can work well when other information is lacking, but be wary of applying population-based statistics too enthusiastically to individual patients.

• *Excessively relying on logical inference.* A real-life example: A patient developed anemia, weakness, and loss of weight. Because he had engaged in high-risk sexual behavior, his physicians at first suspected AIDS, but he was HIV negative. Subsequently, he was diagnosed as having leukemia.

OBSERVING THE MENTAL STATUS

The MSE provides the organizational framework for the observations we use to evaluate and reevaluate the health of our patients. Whether or not you consciously think in terms of the MSE, the observations it comprises should be a familiar part of every mental health clinician's workday. By and large, these observations do not require special questioning or procedures, only an alertness to the information that can be extracted from any ordinary therapy session—for that matter, from any casual conversation. Every time you meet with a patient, you notice aspects of appearance and behavior, speech, content of thought, mood, cognitive status, and insight and judgment—that is, the six traditional parts of the mental status exam.

When you note that a change has occurred in one of these familiar MSE parts, that is the time to begin to wonder why. Of course, it is often the case that such a change is benign and has no importance at all, but the only safe procedure is to consider this comforting possibility last. The other two possible causes for such changes are a primary mental disorder and a physical illness. The safe course is to consider physical causes first, because of the potential for serious, perhaps irreparable harm that can sometimes result when one is treated too late or not at all. Only after it is certain that physical disease has been competently excluded is it safe to assume that the change in MSE symptoms is due to a mental disorder.

In the following pages I will discuss the parts of the MSE, with special emphasis on those observations that may help identify physical disorders. I have grouped the observations into six categories and arranged them in the order that I have used for decades. Of course, any other grouping or order will work just fine, as long as you remember to make all the observations.

In the following discussion I have emphasized those aspects that are likely to convey information about physical disorders. Of course, there are many other symptoms included in the typical MSE; I have focused on those listed here because they are especially likely to be caused by physical disease. Table 3 outlines the complete MSE, including those aspects unlikely to be affected by physical disorders.

TABLE 3. Outline of the Initial Interview

Chief complaint
History of present illness
  Stressors
  Onset
  Symptoms
  Previous episodes
    Treatment
    Consequences
  Course
  Treatment so far
  Hospitalizations?
  Effects on patient,
    others
Personal and social
  Childhood and
    growing up
    Where born
    Number of siblings
      and position
    Reared by both
      parents?
    Relationship with
      parents
    If adopted:
      What
        circumstances?
      Extrafamilial?
  Health as child
  Problems with puberty
  Abuse (physical or
    sexual)
  Education
    Last grade
      completed
    Scholastic problems
    Overly active
    School refusal
    Behavior problems
    Suspension or
      expulsion
  Sociable as child?
  Hobbies?
Life as an adult
  Current living situation:
    Lives with whom?
    Where?
    Ever homeless?
    Support network
    Mobility
    Finances
  Marital
    Age

Number of
  marriages
Number, age, and
  sex of children
Stepchildren?
Marital problems?
Sexual preference,
  adjustment
  Problems with
    intercourse
  Birth control
    methods
  Extramarital
    partners
  Physical, sexual
    abuse?
Work history
  Current occupation
  Number of jobs
  Reasons for job
    changes
  Ever fired?
Leisure activities
  Clubs, organizations
  Interests, hobbies
Military
  Branch, rank
  Years served
  Disciplinary
    problems?
  Combat?
Legal problems ever?
  Criminal
  Litigation
Religion
  Denomination
  Interest
Past medical history
  Major illnesses
  Operations
  Nonpsychiatric
    medications
  Allergies
    Environmental
    Food
    To medications
  Nonmental
    hospitalizations
  Physical impairments
  Risk factors for AIDS?
  Adult physical, sexual
    abuse?

Review of systems
  Disorders of appetite
  Head injury
  Seizures
  Chronic pain
  Unconsciousness
  Premenstrual syndrome
  Review for
    somatization disorder
Family history
  Describe relatives
  Mental disorder in
    relatives
Substance abuse
  Type of substance
  Duration of use
  Quantity
  Consequences
    Medical problems
    Loss of control
    Personal and
      interpersonal
    Job
    Legal
    Financial
  Abuse of medicines
    Prescription
    Over-the-counter
Personality traits
  Lifelong behavior
    patterns
  Violence
  Arrests
Suicide attempts
  Methods
  Consequences
  Drug or alcohol
    associated
  Seriousness
    Psychological
    Physical
Mental status exam
  Appearance
    Apparent age
    Race
    Posture
    Nutrition
    Hygiene
    Hairstyle
    Clothing
      Neat?
      Clean?

(continued)

Fashion	Content of thought	Person
Behavior	Phobias	Place
Activity level	Anxiety	Time
Tremors?	Obsessions and	Memory
Mannerisms and	compulsions	Immediate
stereotypies	Thoughts of suicide	Recent
Smiles?	Delusions	Remote
Eye contact	Hallucinations	Attention and
Speaks with accent?	Language	concentration
Mood	Comprehension	Serial sevens
Type	Fluency	Count backward
Lability	Naming	Cultural information
Appropriateness	Repetition	Five presidents
Flow of thought	Reading	Abstract thinking
Word associations	Writing	Similarities
Rate and rhythm of	Cognitive	Differences
speech	Orientation	

Note. From Morrison, James: *The First Interview: Revised for DSM-IV.* New York: Guilford Press, 1995, p. 8. Copyright 1995 by The Guilford Press. Reprinted by permission.

In the following pages, I have discussed the MSE as it relates to physical disease. The disorders listed in **boldface** are those discussed in this book that may be suggested by particular MSE findings. For a fuller discussion of performing and evaluating the complete MSE, see suggested readings in the Appendix.

APPEARANCE AND BEHAVIOR

Alertness

If your patient is not fully alert, what description seems appropriate? Wandering attention often indicates delirium, a rapid cognitive decline with reduced level of consciousness. Delirium can have a whole host of causes—circulatory, deficiency (such as vitamins or minerals), endocrine, infectious, metabolic, neoplastic, or traumatic. Patients with **liver failure** will sometimes fall asleep, even in the middle of a conversation. Fluctuating levels of alertness may also be found in patients suffering from **chronic obstructive lung disease**. (But be careful: Someone who is merely hard of hearing might give a false appearance of inattention.)

By the time of his disability exam, John Elmore had about given up. For nearly a year his memory seemed to be failing him. Although he was only 57, it seemed to all who knew him that he was developing Alzheimer's. His mood had been low. Though at one time he took medication for a possible depressive pseudodementia, it didn't much affect his overall clinical condition. Besides his memory, he complained of trouble focusing attention, and coworkers noted that he occasionally fell asleep while seated in front of his computer screen.

Close questioning at a workers' compensation exam revealed that months earlier, while trying out his grandson's skateboard in the garage, John had fallen and struck his head.

"I didn't think it was very important," he admitted. "I told myself I was only dazed, but I guess I could have been out for a minute or two. It was pretty embarrassing, so I never told anyone."

An MRI of his head revealed a small **subdural hematoma**.

Attitude toward Examiner

Is your patient friendly or reserved? Hostile or suspicious? Apparent apathy suggests that your patient finds the conversation boring or, at any rate, less compelling than other subjects. Or does the apathy instead simply indicate tiredness, which can be a symptom of many disorders including **protein energy malnutrition**, **fibromyalgia**, **hypertension**, **multiple sclerosis**, **premenstrual syndrome**, and **systemic lupus erythematosus**, to name a few.

> For a time, a psychiatrist thought that he needed psychiatric help himself. "It got to the point that I didn't have much interest in my patients. I didn't even want to get up in the morning."
>
> Fortunately, when he finally sought help it was from his internist. Although he couldn't remember the tick bite, he tested positive for **Lyme disease**. A course of antibiotics rapidly restored his interest in work.

Here, as in every other aspect of the MSE, it is important to keep alert for changes from the patient's usual behavior. It is especially important in ongoing therapy that the clinician remain alert for sudden shifts of attitude—a flare-up of hostility, an unwonted lapse of attention—that could suggest the development of a new disease process.

Age

What is your patient's apparent age, and how does it compare with chronological age? Serious, especially chronic, physical illness such as heart disease leaves its mark on people's faces, making them seem older than their years. Remember that being overweight, whether due to simple obesity or to more exotic causes such as **Cushing's disease**, fills out wrinkles, often giving the patient a youthful look. Try to discern the patient's true age beneath the camouflage afforded by a beard or wig.

Posture

Notice your patient's posture; is it stooped, as with **parkinsonism**? Hunched from collapsed vertebrae (this may be caused by osteoporosis from **hyperparathyroidism**)? Even a ramrod-straight bearing should not escape your attention—is it the product of a long military career or a spinal fusion?

Body Build

How would you describe body build? Athletic? If heavyset or obese, could this be due to **hypothyroidism**? (Remember that obese patients are also at risk for **sleep apnea**.) Slender? A patient who is thin to the point of gauntness could have anorexia nervosa, but might instead have a physical disease such as **diabetes, hyperthyroidism**, or **protein energy malnutrition**.

> Sitting there in the waiting room, Barry Olden didn't look much different from the other two prison inmates. But when he stood up for his appointment, the clinician who had called him in made a couple of observations.
>
> "He got up, and then it seemed like he just kept on getting up," she said. "But it wasn't just that he was tall. It

was his proportions. His belt buckle was higher than the middle of his body. Most of his 6'7" was legs!"

A genetic study later revealed that Barry had an extra X chromosome, 47 chromosomes in all, leading to a diagnosis of **Klinefelter's syndrome**.

General Motor Activity

Is your patient either underactive or overactive? An unusually low degree of motor activity may be associated with conditions as diverse as **hypothyroidism** and **fibromyalgia**.

On the other side of the activity spectrum is fidgetiness, which could express simple anxiety. However, could it instead be an early expression of **Huntington's disease**? Is the patient who appears agitated merely worried about something, or are anxiety and agitation both precipitated by **chronic obstructive lung disease**? Could this be an agitated delirium, perhaps caused by **hyperparathyroidism**?

> In her first visit to the therapist, Henrietta Dockery literally paced the floor. "Of course I'm nervous! I've got four kids under the age of 5—nervous is what I'm paid for! My God, it's hot in here."
>
> Her husband chimed in, "Sure, you've always been anxious. But now you're agitated. You haven't sat still for 2 minutes since we got here."
>
> Henrietta's eyes widened a little further than usual, and she tried to open the collar of a blouse that seemed too lightweight for February. Her therapist thought that her neck looked somewhat fuller than would be expected for a slender woman still in her 20s and referred her for a medical checkup. The answer came back **hyperthyroidism**, unsurprising in view of the number of typical symptoms.

Akathisia is a special form of motor overactivity in which the patient feels incapable of sitting still and must repeatedly get up and move about the room. It usually indicates the side effect of a neuroleptic drug, but it can also occur in patients with dementia.

Watch for evidence of apraxia, that is, difficulty your patient might have accomplishing ordinary tasks—clumsiness in buttoning a coat, writing—despite the absence of evidence of any physical weakness. Apraxias suggest a serious neurological disorder such as a **stroke** or **Alzheimer's disease**.

> Elisabeth Seeley had first sought supportive psychotherapy nearly a year earlier, following the death of her husband of 45 years. Every other week for months, she had sat, carefully dressed and not a hair out of place, matching purse held primly on her lap, while discussing her loneliness.
>
> But over the past several sessions, a change had become evident. Her first symptom had been a series of mismatched purses; more recently, she had appeared downright untidy—usually rumpled, once with a spot of scrambled egg stuck to the placket of her blouse. When putting her coat on, she seemed unable to get even the large buttons into their holes.
>
> After totaling the results of a Mini-Mental State Exam (MMSE), her therapist requested a dementia workup.

Catatonic symptoms, abnormalities of motility, first comprehensively described in 1874, are uncommon today even in large mental hospitals. These symptoms include, among others, catalepsy (the patient holds an abnormal posture, despite being told to relax it), waxy flexibility (resistance to passive bending of a limb), negativism (resistance to a command), mutism, and stereotypies (purposeless, repetitive movements). Although they have traditionally been associated with schizophrenia and mood disorders, they have also been reported in such diverse conditions as **epilepsy**, **tuberous sclerosis**, **thiamine deficiency**, and at least one form of **homocystinuria**.

> When the paramedics found him, he was sitting in a doorway, dazed and mute. He resisted their attempts at examination, tightly closing his eyes when asked to open them. So he was admitted as "John Doe" to the hospital's locked unit, where the following morning a nursing aide made a discovery.
>
> "He was just lying there on his back, still as a rock, and I wanted to do something for him. I started to fluff his pillow, but when I removed it, his head didn't move. I mean, it just sort of hung there, suspended in midair, an inch or two above the mattress. He's still that way now, and it's been 5 minutes!"

Someone suggested schizophrenia, but the consultant pointed out that catatonic schizophrenia was uncommon and that there were numerous physical causes that could explain catatonic symptoms. Routine laboratory testing quickly found evidence suggesting **hyperparathyroidism**.

Gait

When your patient arises from a chair in the waiting room and walks across the floor to greet you, take the opportunity to make observations about general body movement. Are the body motions smooth and graceful? Unsteady or halting gait suggests a variety of medical and neurological problems including **liver failure**, **normal pressure hydrocephalus**, **cerebral ataxia**, **Creutzfeldt–Jakob disease**, and **progressive supranuclear palsy**.

Herb Gorman had last appeared at the clinic 2 years earlier for several sessions of predivorce counseling. After the last of these, Herb declared himself "free as a bird" and, almost literally, skipped out of the office into the arms of soon-to-be wife number three.

Now he was back, complaining of depression, and he definitely wasn't skipping. "If anything, he schleps," Herb's clinician told the consulting neurologist on the telephone. "In fact, that's what I noticed most about him—those tiny, shuffling steps he took. And now he doesn't seem to have any affect at all. He's just about totally expressionless."

That same day, the clinician's impression of **Parkinson's disease** was confirmed.

Tremor

Tremor (shakiness, usually seen in the upper extremities) may take any of several forms. In a coarse tremor, such as occurs when a person withdraws from heavy alcohol use, the shaking is so obvious that you'll notice it from across the room; the patient may be even unable to drink from a glass of water without spilling. However, a fine tremor may be so subtle that, to be seen, it must be amplified by a note card placed on the backs of the patient's fingers as they are spread in midair.

An intention tremor is one that appears only when the patient tries to carry out hand movements such as touching a forefinger precisely to a spot on a piece of paper. The finger shakes coarsely as it approaches and often misses the spot, suggesting a diagnosis such as **brain injury** or **multiple sclerosis**. Pill-rolling tremor—the back-and-forth motion of the thumb against index and middle fingers, as if rubbing them together— occurs mainly when the hand is at rest. It is found in **Parkinson's disease** or pseudoparkinsonism induced by neuroleptic drugs. Finally, fine tremor may indicate **thyroid disease**, **low blood sugar**, anxiety, or the use of medications such as lithium or antidepressants.

> As an insulin-dependent diabetic, psychotherapist Leslie Kaye was unusually alert for symptoms of the disease in others. Twice during office visits, patients had presented with symptoms that suggested the need for better control of their own diabetes.
> Recently, Louise, a teenager who had been taking insulin for only about 4 months, had complained of anxiety, and her hand had shaken so badly that she had spilled her can of diet soda. Suspecting an insulin reaction, Leslie substituted orange juice for the diet drink and referred Louise back to the endocrinologist for another medication adjustment.

Another sort of tremor, coarser but rarer than any of those just mentioned, is that which occurs in **Wilson's disease**. The entire upper arm will flap at the shoulder, and if the patient's arm is bent at the elbow, the effect resembles the beating of a bird's wing. Asterixis is a coarse tremor of the outstretched hand at the wrist. It is found in patients with end-stage **liver failure**.

Finally, keep in mind that some people have inherited a condition called benign or familial tremor. It is frequently encountered (around 1 in every 200 people in the general population). It may appear at its worst during stress and may only be noticed when the arms are outstretched. Although these individuals are sometimes misdiagnosed as having parkinsonism, benign tremor is usually just that: benign.

The same therapist had referred Jerrold Pontius to a neurologist. Jerrold had just begun treatment for "self-actualization," and during a portion of the initial psychological testing his hand shook so badly that he could not write a sentence from dictation. After the neurologist made a diagnosis of benign tremor, Jerrold and the therapist had a discussion about symptoms and the "worried well."

Tardive Dyskinesia (TD)

These abnormal movements of the face and shoulders develop after prolonged exposure to neuroleptic drugs such as chlorpromazine. The movements may be obvious (repeated protrusion of the tongue or pursing of lips) or subtle (rhythmic motions of the tongue only when it is at rest inside the mouth). The risk of TD is greater with higher dose, longer exposure, and in patients who do not have schizophrenia.

Facial Expression

Notice the degree to which your patient's expression changes as you converse. Although schizophrenia may cause a fixed, unchanging expression, also consider the possibility of a facial paralysis due to **Lyme disease** or **Parkinson's disease**. (The paralysis caused by Bell's palsy is usually unilateral and is not associated with mental or behavioral symptoms.)

Involuntary contractions, or spasms, of the face are most likely caused by tics, but facial grimacing can also be a symptom of **hypoparathyroidism**.

Gaze

A strong, steady gaze probably means that the other person is interested in what you have to say, but could it denote a neurological disorder such as **parkinsonism**? A patient who cannot look downward may be suffering from **progressive supranuclear palsy**. Nystagmus, the rapid flickering of the gaze back and forth (sometimes up and down), can be a congenital disorder with no adverse health implications, but it can also be found in disorders as diverse as **thiamine deficiency**, use of sedative drugs, **brain abscess**, and **Ménière's syndrome**.

Warren Oates leaned his cane against the desk in the tiny examining office and sank onto the folding chair. He had just spent 8 hours at the general hospital next door, shuttling from one department to another: general medicine to orthopedics to ophthalmology and back. In the last of these, he had been told to come back in 5 months, their first available appointment. An advice nurse had finally suggested that his problems might be emotional—he had been depressed, after all—and off he was sent to mental health.

There the clinician took down the details of his depression and asked about the cane. Warren explained in halting words that he had limped ever since he could remember, though he thought he had had more difficulty with it recently. As he talked, his gaze seemed to flick back and forth in a subtle, yet definite nystagmus. Suspecting **multiple sclerosis**, the clinician arranged for an emergency appointment with neurology.

Patients with **hyperthyroidism** will sometimes develop exophthalmos, a condition in which the eyeballs appear to protrude farther than normal from their sockets. Hyperthyroid patients will also sometimes have lid lag, a condition in which, with downward gaze, the upper eyelid does *not* fall almost instantly, as is normal. While you are at it, pause to consider what evidence sunglasses worn indoors might conceal—red eyes (marijuana use)? Pupils that are dilated (history of **stroke**, anoxia)? Pinpoint pupils (opioid intoxication)? Or simple tearfulness?

Skin

Unusually dark skin coloring may signify more than just lying in the sun. Be aware of the possibility of **pellagra** or **Addison's disease**. Of course, unusual pallor suggests anemia, but what is the cause—**hypothyroidism**? **Kidney failure**?

"Well, of *course* they're different." Bonnie McCloud was trying to explain the ringing in her ears to her longtime therapist. "The voices are just behind me, and for years I've been able to make them go away if I just take enough medicine. Don't like it though. But the ringing actually sounds in my *ears*, and I've only noticed it for the past few months."

Her therapist noted that she seemed paler than usual. "I know," said Bonnie. "One of my spirit voices has been saying the same thing."

A routine complete blood count pointed to a macrocytic anemia; further testing quickly confirmed the diagnosis of **pernicious anemia**.

Does marked flushing suggest **menopause**? Sudden flushing (or blushing) could be a symptom of social phobia, but it also is characteristic of **carcinoid syndrome**.

Jaundice (abnormal yellow color of the skin, often first noticeable in the whites of the eyes) indicates liver disease. When **liver failure** becomes severe, skin will itch, and patients will scratch.

Some of the grosser skin conditions are pretty evident—the fluid-filled vesicles of **neurofibromatosis**, for example, or the purple blotches of **Sturge–Weber** disease. Rashes are so often benign (think of prickly heat) that you may overlook even some that suggest classical skin pathology.

For several months subsequent to the birth of her third child, Rhoda Barr had complained of depression and fatigue. She, her husband, and their family physician all agreed that she probably had chronic fatigue syndrome, which was how she came to be referred for therapy.

As they began their weekly appointment one afternoon in mid-July, Rhoda's therapist was startled by one aspect of her appearance: She had a bright red rash that spilled across the bridge of her nose onto both cheeks. When questioned, she responded, "It's been so much worse since I've been going to the beach. I used to be able to cover it with makeup, but I finally just gave up."

The consultation revealed the cause of her rash and the fatigue: **systemic lupus erythematosus**.

As you shake hands you may notice either excessive dryness or moisture, which may indicate **hypothyroidism** or **hyperthyroidism**, respectively. Notice any bruises. Although their cause could be benign (simple clumsiness or taking a little too much aspirin), there could instead be ominous implications (physical abuse or **kidney failure** or **liver failure**).

The shape and location of any scars may carry important information: wrist (suicide attempts)? round burns on the extremities from cigarettes (physical abuse or self-mutilation)? surgical half-moon around the front of the neck (thyroidectomy, suggesting the possibility of surgical **hypothyroidism**)?

> While interviewing a patient for an oral board examination, a psychiatrist came to grief. Intent upon taking notes, Dr. Voner failed to notice the small, round scar, partly covered by a lock of hair, on the right side of the patient's forehead. An intense review of those notes that began the instant the interview was over prevented the candidate from noticing the slight limp as the patient departed the room. It was left to the two examiners to suggest one possible conclusion: This depressed patient was in fact a survivor of a self-administered gunshot wound that had not been disclosed during the course of the interview.

Hair

What can you notice about the hair, the skin's principal appendage? Of course, half of all adults normally experience hair loss, but in either sex, it could be due to **liver failure** or **malnutrition**. Increased body hair (this will be most noticeable in women) suggests endocrine disease such as a tumor of an adrenal gland or **liver failure**. Patients with **hyperthyroidism** sometimes note that their hair has become finer (meaning a decreased diameter) than it once was.

> When Naomi Hershey appeared for her screening appointment during National Depression Awareness Week, almost the first thing the clinician noticed was her hair. It looked dull and sparse, and the outer portion of each eyebrow appeared to be missing entirely. Laboratory testing revealed **hypothyroidism**.

Odors

Notice any unusual odors. Of course, bad breath is most likely due to inadequate oral hygiene, but it can be the product of **liver failure** (fetor hepaticus). The smell of urine about the clothing suggests incontinence, one cause of which can be **normal pressure hydrocephalus**.

Clothing

Is clothing clean, neat, and appropriate to the climate? There is much that clinicians infer (not always accurately) about social background, economic circumstances, and diagnosis of mental disorder from clothing that is tattered, dirty, skimpy, or inappropriate to temperature. Dementia of various causes may be hinted at by untidy grooming or clothing: breakfast spilled across a shirtfront, buttons misbuttoned, an absent sock, or untied shoe.

> Eleanor Townsend wasn't sure why she was seeking help. She had been healthy all her adult life, through the rearing of four children and a subsequent "mini-career" as a writer of children's fiction. Now she didn't really feel ill, so she hadn't consulted her family doctor. But she hadn't felt exactly well, either—perhaps a little depressed, which was why she had sought therapy.
>
> Eleanor looked bright and cheerful. In fact, her mental status seemed completely normal, with one exception: Her carefully pressed white skirt was marred by a streak of paint that ran across her left hip. It was suspiciously like a freshly painted railing that the therapist had noted outside the office upon returning from lunch that day. Eleanor could not remember running into anything, but on close questioning she admitted to several other unaccountable instances of mussed clothing or finding herself someplace she hadn't meant to go. Subsequently, an electroencephalogram (EEG) showed abnormal activity in the right temporal lobe, and magnetic resonance imaging (MRI) revealed a tumor that proved to be a **meningioma**.

Voice

Has the pitch of your patient's voice changed since you have been acquainted? Lower pitch or hoarseness can result from cigarette smoking, but **hypothyroidism** is another possibility.

An elderly man shot and killed his landlady, whom he thought had organized a plot against him. The origin of his psychosis was ultimately traced to a **brain tumor** that had metastasized from his lung. The clue to this diagnosis was provided by his voice, which had recently become high-pitched and gravelly, probably due to a vocal cord paralyzed by the primary tumor.

Other Items of Appearance and Behavior

Ankle swelling (edema) suggests several physical disorders including **congestive heart failure**, **premenstrual syndrome**, and **thiamine deficiency**.

Watch for any other peculiar sorts of behavior.

- **Diabetes mellitus** was diagnosed in a hospitalized patient when staff noted that he was saving each of the Styrofoam cups from which he drank—dozens of them each day, indicating profound thirst.
- Another patient, chronically hospitalized for schizophrenia, was noted to spend much of his day at the water fountain. He was investigated for symptoms of **encephalopathy** caused by low blood sodium (hyponatremia).

However, remember that not all unusual behavior signifies a physical disorder:

- Whenever staff members were present, a patient would try to obtain Artane by pacing the room with his neck twisted and eyes rolled ceiling ward, imitating acute dystonia.

MOOD (AFFECT)

Although these terms are often used interchangeably, *affect* usually indicates not only a statement of feeling (*mood*) but also physical features (facial expression, activity level) that indicate how the patient *appears* to be feeling. The three dimensions of mood to watch for include type, lability, and appropriateness.

Type of Mood

Mood *type* is an expression of the patient's current emotional state. It is expressed as an adjective that completes the statement, "I feel. . . . " Although there are dozens of words we can use to express how we feel, they can be reduced to the following basic categories: anger, anxiety, contentment, disgust, fear, guilt, irritation, joy, sadness, shame, and surprise. Several of these are often associated with physical illness.

Sadness (Depression)

Of course, the fact of having any serious illness is inherently depressing, but I refer here to something more than just the reaction to bad news. The illnesses discussed below are thought capable of physiologically producing symptoms of depression, even in patients who may be unaware that they have a medical illness. Of course, the patient's experience is likely to include far more that just sadness. Rather, the symptom of depression will often be accompanied by other symptoms of major depressive episode, including fatigue, guilt, poor concentration, thoughts of death, loss of interest and appetite, increased or decreased psychomotor activity, and changes (increase or decrease) in sleep, appetite, and weight.

Up to half of patients with seizure disorders (**epilepsy**) may have depressive symptoms, whereas the percentage for **diabetes** approaches two-thirds. Four other endocrine disorders that may cause depression are **hypothyroidism, hyperthyroidism, hypoparathyroidism**, and **hyperparathyroidism**. Depression can also result from changes in the physical architecture of the brain produced by **multiple sclerosis, stroke**, and **brain trauma**. Metabolic disorders include **porphyria** and **Wilson's disease**. Infectious diseases include **Lyme disease** and **syphilis**. At least one vitamin deficiency (**pellagra**) has been implicated, as has the inherited neurological disorder **Huntington's disease**. Two others are **Parkinson's disease** and **cancer of the pancreas**. Several examples are cited throughout this section.

Anxiety

As you might imagine, anxiety symptoms, including panic attacks, have been related to a variety of disorders that affect the functioning of heart or lungs, including **lung cancer**, **mitral valve prolapse**, **cardiac arrhythmias**, and **chronic obstructive lung disease**.

> At age 45, Breffni O'Connell was being treated for seasonal mood disorder. Regularly for 10 years, he had felt depressed each November, resulting in feelings of guilt (about the failure of his marriage, imagined failures at work, the mental retardation of his oldest son), anxiety attacks, and even suicidal ideas. Antidepressant medication invariably helped his low moods and anxiety, but it wasn't until spring of each succeeding year that his mood truly lightened and he became, in his words, "A little hyper."
>
> After years of these cycles, one May morning he awakened to "the worst panic attack I ever had." He felt that he could not get his breath and sat panting by an open window: "Just trying to wring enough oxygen out of the air." Although he denied he felt depressed ("Just scared"), he restarted his antidepressants. Over the next several days, his sleep remained disturbed, his appetite plummeted, and his anxiety and agitation increased to the point that he paced the house and hyperventilated.
>
> When he could no longer tolerate the constant fear that he might die, he was admitted to the hospital. Physical exam revealed bubbling noises in his chest when he took a deep breath; a chest X-ray confirmed pneumonia. The antidepressants were stopped and antibiotics started. Within 3 days, the anxiety attacks had disappeared, and he was breathing normally.

But panic attacks have also been reported in complaints not directly referable to the chest, including **Ménière's syndrome**, insulin reactions in **diabetes**, and **fibromyalgia**. Other anxiety symptoms have been noted in disorders as diverse as **hyperparathyroidism**, **hyperthyroidism**, **Lyme disease**, **anemia**, **pheochromocytoma**, **porphyria**, and **premenstrual syndrome**. The sense of impending doom often noted in panic disorder may also be reported by patients bleeding from the gastrointestinal tract.

Irritability

The literature mentions a few medical disorders specifically associated with this affect: **hyperthyroidism**, **migraine**, **sleep**

apnea, and the **syndrome of inappropriate ADH secretion**. Undoubtedly, however, there are others.

Joy (Euphoria)

An undue degree of elation is an occasional feature of **Huntington's disease**, **multiple sclerosis**, **stroke**, and other causes of **brain injury** (such as contusion).

Lability of Mood

It can be entirely normal for a person to go from laughter to tears, and back again, within a relatively short period of time. After all, who has not had this experience while watching a movie or reading a book? But excessive lability of mood that occurs without much provocation can be found in **liver failure**, **multiple sclerosis**, **Creutzfeldt–Jakob disease**, **strokes**, and **progressive supranuclear palsy**.

At the other extreme is emotional blunting (reduced lability), classically associated with schizophrenia but also found as a feature of dementia. Facial immobility (some refer to it as flattening of mood) may cause the affect of patients with **Parkinson's disease** to appear stiff or frozen, but this appearance belies their true feelings.

Appropriateness of Mood

The third quality of mood is its appropriateness to the content of what is being thought or said. A patient who laughs at the death of a parent may be showing inappropriateness of affect. (Of course, you would have to know all the facts—the parent might have been a tyrant.) Inappropriate emotion, while often attributable to schizophrenia, is found in a condition called pseudobulbar palsy, which can be a symptom of conditions such as **stroke** and **multiple sclerosis**.

During one therapy session Rowena Palmer wondered aloud about her mother's behavior. "I'll tell her something sad or maybe something that's irritated me. And often, she'll just laugh. She's so perverse. I sometimes think she's just trying to get under my skin."

Recalling the mother's recent stroke, the therapist suggested that the behavior could be actually caused by her neurological condition, not her personality.

SPEECH

Abnormalities of flow of speech, which often mirror abnormal flow of thought, can be divided into two principal types: problems with rate and rhythm of speech, and problems with the coherence of speech (the way thoughts are joined together).

Rate and Rhythm

Rate of Speech

The rate at which most people talk ranges from about 140–160 words per minute—around five syllables per second. Rates outside either end of that range we usually associate with mental disorder, such as schizophrenia, major depression, and mania. But speech that is abnormally rapid may be due to metabolic problems such as **hyperthyroidism**, and complete muteness may be due to a variety of conditions that include **brain tumors**, **stroke**, and **Huntington's disease**.

Abnormal Speech Rhythm

Rhythm of speech (in essence, the regularity of spacing between words) can be affected by a variety of neurological conditions. The most common of these is **multiple sclerosis**, in which every few words, the speaker interjects a pause into the flow of speech. This results in a sing-song quality that is sometimes called scanning speech. The much less common **Wilson's disease** can produce difficulty speaking or swallowing.

Also note any lack of clarity of speech. Of course, mumbling can be due to habit, and slurring of words can be caused by simple intoxication, but be alert for other causes of recent changes in the patient's speech clarity. These might include

stroke, progressive neuromuscular diseases such as **multiple sclerosis**, and the effects of low blood sugar, such as might be found in poorly controlled **diabetes mellitus**.

> Because Humphrey Cottrell had faithfully attended Alcoholics Anonymous for 25 years, his therapist was surprised to observe during several midmorning sessions that Humphrey had begun to slur his words. Upon discussion, Humphrey revealed that he had been having difficulty controlling his diabetes. He resolved to work harder on his diet and to pay another visit to his endocrinologist.

Coherence of Speech

Here is an area of the MSE that is dominated by the functional mental disorders. Notice how your patient ties thoughts together into a stream. Does one idea logically follow its predecessor, or do you have difficulty understanding the relationship between consecutive ideas?

Speech that includes successive ideas that are logically unrelated and in a context in which the listener cannot perceive the intention behind the speaker's thought processes is referred to as tangential speech, and the actual skip from one thought to another is referred to as a derailment. (Minor example: "I guess I'll stay awhile and strap on a bookmobile.") As you might imagine, derailments can vary in their severity and must be distinguished from thought patterns that are inattentive or intentionally humorous or poetic. Tangential speech must also be distinguished from that which is merely circumstantial. A circumstantial patient may consume unnecessary time and words, introducing any number of extraneous topics, some more related than others, before eventually, much like this sentence, rambling back to the point. Such discursive speech, while unfocused and tedious, is seldom pathological.

Pathological derailment, indicating a disorder of the form of thought, usually results from an endogenous psychosis such as schizophrenia or bipolar disorder. Even more extreme degrees of formal thought disorder—word salad, in which the patient speaks words or phrases that bear no apparent relation to one another and convey no sense of organized thought whatsoever—may be encountered in severe neurological disorders. Such speech is rare and unlikely to be encountered, even in a mental health practitioner's office.

CONTENT OF THOUGHT

Hallucinations

Affecting any of the five senses, hallucinations occur when patients perceive sensation in the absence of actual stimulus. The most common type, the auditory hallucination, nearly always indicates a "functional" psychosis such as schizophrenia or manic–depressive illness.

Occasionally, a patient with severe alcoholism will develop auditory hallucinations shortly after the drinking stops. This condition, the symptoms of which closely resemble paranoid schizophrenia, used to be called alcoholic auditory hallucinosis. In DSM-IV it has been renamed alcohol-induced psychotic disorder, with hallucinations,* which uses a few additional words to convey only a little less information.

On the other hand, hallucinations of other senses, especially those that develop relatively rapidly, are much more likely than auditory hallucinations to be caused by general medical illnesses. For example, **stroke** patients may perceive light, shape, or formed objects in the absence of any actual visual stimulus. These images may change when the patient blinks. **Epilepsy** patients may experience hallucinations of sight, smell, or taste as the aura that warns them they are about to have a seizure. Hallucinations of one sort or another have been sporadically reported in a wide variety of other medical conditions, including **Huntington's disease, hyperparathyroidism** and **hypoparathyroidism, kidney failure, syphilis**, and **Wilson's disease**.

> For most of his adult life, Johnnie Norwood had heard two voices. One told him that he was the "Lamb of God," the other, that he was "The Antichrist." After years combating the forces of good and evil, he finally gave up the struggle

*Not the same as the visual hallucinations of the far more common alcohol withdrawal.

and, for the last two decades, had dwelled on a mental ward in a Veterans Administration hospital.

Johnnie celebrated his 65th birthday by announcing "the Triumph of the Righteous, I've seen the light." The light he had seen was literal. For several weeks, he had been hallucinating flashing lights that appeared on the right side of his visual fields. "It feels like I'm living inside a video game," he commented. When an increase in his antipsychotic medication made no difference, a medical consultation was requested. Ultimately, the diagnosis of **porphyria** was made.

Hallucinations must always be carefully discriminated from illusions. Whereas a hallucination is a wholly made-up experience, an illusion is based upon a sensory experience that the patient misinterprets. The actual sensory stimulus may be one that is poorly perceived. For example, in a dark room, lighted only by the flickering glow of a small television, a child's jump rope is briefly seen as a huge, coiled snake. Fleeting and readily corrected with better lighting or a second glance, illusions are both commonplace and nonpathological.

Delusions

A delusion is a false belief that cannot be shaken and is not in keeping with the patient's cultural background. Delusions may be encountered in some of the same illnesses just mentioned; they are especially common in dementia. Certain types of delusions may have specific diagnostic import. Patients with **epilepsy** are especially likely to develop persecutory delusions; alcoholic patients may believe that a spouse has become unfaithful (delusions of infidelity).

On her honeymoon, Wanda Teller experienced her first-ever psychomotor seizure. Already 3 months pregnant, she refused to take medication until her twin daughters were safely delivered. Since then, she had continued to have a seizure once or twice a year, just often enough to keep her from driving but not enough to interfere with the rest of her life.

Now that the girls were nearly grown, she was seeking therapy to determine how to relate to them. "They're not mine," she explained. "They look just the same, but someone replaced them."

Eventually, delusional disorder (with Capgras delusions) and **temporal lobe epilepsy** were diagnosed.

From delusions discriminate depersonalization, which is the persistent feeling that the individual has changed, and derealization, the persistent feeling that the environment has changed. Also note any experiences the patient may report of *déjà vu* (French for "already seen"), the feeling of having experienced or seen a particular situation before, when such is probably not the case. *Déjà vu* is an extremely common experience that most of us have probably had at one time or another. However, it can sometimes be a symptom of **temporal lobe epilepsy**. In the conditions described in this paragraph, the beliefs are held with much less intensity than is true of delusions; that is, if pressed, the patient will readily admit that the environment has not really changed, that this could be the first time for a particular experience, and so forth.

Violence and Suicidal Ideas

Violence

A history of violent behavior is especially associated with personality disorder (especially antisocial and borderline) and some Axis I disorders as well (schizophrenia, mania, intermittent explosive disorder, mental retardation). But violent behavior has also been reported in some physical disorders—**epilepsy** (either during the seizure or between seizures), **brain infections** (syphilis, fungal infections, herpes), and in a broad variety of other central nervous system and general medical disorders that include **normal pressure hydrocephalus, brain trauma, stroke, multiple sclerosis,** and **Alzheimer's, Huntington's, Parkinson's,** and **Wilson's diseases.** Other disorders occasionally associated with violence include **Cushing's disease, electrolyte imbalance, hyperthyroidism, hypothyroidism, liver disease, porphyria, renal disease, systemic infections, systemic lupus erythematosus,** some vitamin deficiencies, and various causes of low blood sugar.

Patients seldom volunteer information about violent behavior. But it is so important that it must be carefully inquired after in any patient for whom aggressive–hostile or otherwise violent behavior seems a possibility.

Suicidal Behaviors

Frequently encountered in a mental health population are suicidal ideas and behaviors. They must be sought in every new mental health patient interviewed. Of course, suicide is not specific to any one mental or physical diagnosis, but rather is behavior that can be found in nearly any mental health diagnosis and a wide variety of physical disorders.

Among medical patients, as in mental patients, the most important guidepost to ultimate suicidal activity may be provided by demographics and the specifics of the individual's situation. A number of demographic and other characteristics make up the profile of the typical suicidal patient:

- Old age
- Male sex
- Living alone
- No emotional support
- Terminal illness (real or imagined)
- Severe pain
- Use of drugs or alcohol
- Lack of employment
- Depressive episode (in either major depressive disorder or bipolar mood disorder)
- Schizophrenia

Those thoughts aside, the physical disorders that have been especially linked to completed suicide include **cancer** of any type, **epilepsy**, **Huntington's disease**, and **kidney failure**.

Other Thought Content

An obsession is a belief, idea, or thought that persistently dominates the patient's thought content, despite the fact that the patient recognizes that it is unrealistic and may try to resist it.

A compulsion is an act that is performed repeatedly, in such a way that the patient realizes it is neither appropriate nor useful. A phobia is an unreasonable, intense fear associated with some object or situation. Obsessions and phobias are not usually caused by physical disease, but they have been reported with **hypoparathyroidism**; obsessions have been associated with **Lyme disease**.

Of course, the thought content of most patients is likely to include none of these marks of psychopathology. Rather, what most patients talk about is the stuff of everyday life: jobs, relationships, hopes, dreams, current events—and health. Because all sorts of patients are likely to discuss physical health concerns with their mental health providers, the best clue to physical disease may be some very direct statement ("I've noticed a lump under my arm," "My clothing doesn't seem so loose, anymore," or "I think my memory's shot"). Of course, any such statement indicating a change in physical health status should be noted and its implications for action carefully considered.

INTELLECTUAL RESOURCES

In this section of the MSE especially, it is valuable to have baseline information against which to gauge new findings. Here is an undeniable reason for performing, and carefully recording, a formal MSE on every patient.

Attention and Concentration

Attention is defined as the ability to focus on a current topic or task, whereas concentration is the ability to sustain that focus over a longer period of time. Your patient's behavior throughout the course of the interview is the best way to judge attention and concentration. If you need additional evidence, ask the patient to subtract serial sevens, stopping at, say, 27. If this task is too difficult, try serial threes or counting backward by ones.

Each of these calculation tasks really tests attention and may be abnormal in disorders as diverse as **fibromyalgia** and **postconcussion syndrome**, plus a variety of disorders that produce delirium. Among the causes of delirium detailed in this book are **cancer** (systemic and brain), **cardiac arrhythmia**, **chronic obstructive lung disease**, **hypertensive encephalopathy**, **hyperparathyroidism**, **hypoparathyroidism**, **inappropriate ADH secretion**, **liver failure**, **normal pressure hydrocephalus**, **hypothyroidism**, **multiple sclerosis**, **pellagra**, **postoperative states**, **stroke**, **subdural hematoma**, **systemic infection**, **thiamine deficiency**, and **Wilson's**, **Huntington's**, and **Creutzfeldt–Jakob diseases**.

Orientation

You might think it would be obvious when a patient is disoriented for person, place, or time, but some patients become skilled at hiding embarrassing defects of memory. To be certain, you may have to ask. In cognitive disorders, orientation to time (allow a day or two as the leeway any normal person might require) usually goes first, followed by place. Disorientation that extends to personal identity is decidedly unusual. Even a mild degree of disorientation may point to any of the many possible causes of cognitive disorder listed previously, as well as to a substance-related disorder, Alzheimer's disease, or vascular dementia.

Language

The assessment of the patient's language capabilities can be broken down into several parts:

- *Comprehension* of a spoken directive.
- *Fluency,* or the ability to use normal vocabulary and prosody to construct sentences of normal length.
- *Naming* of everyday objects without resorting to circumlocutions such as "A thing to write with" for a pencil.
- *Repetition* of a standard phrase such as "No ifs, ands, or buts."
- *Reading* a sentence or two from a page.
- *Writing* a sentence from dictation.

Abnormalities of any of these language functions may indicate stroke, or any of the causes of delirium or dementia listed previously.

Memory

Problems with memory may become evident in several ways:

- *Encoding and immediate recall.* The patient cannot repeat words or numbers presented by the examiner seconds earlier.
- *Short-term memory.* The patient cannot recall, for example, a list of three words (such as a color, a name, and a street address) several minutes after the initial presentation.
- *Long-term memory.* The patient has difficulty recalling information learned long ago—dates of marriage, births of children, or even the names of siblings.

Any problem with memory suggests a possible cognitive disorder, especially one of the dementias, although other causes of inattention (delirium, anxiety, "pseudodementia" due to depression) must also be considered. Even patients with a dementia as severe as Alzheimer's will retain long-term memories better than short-term memories. But with progression of the disease, even information learned in childhood will eventually be lost.

> When Rollie Andersen had to perform the tasks just listed as a part of the MMSE, he scored a discouraging 18 out of a possible 30. Among his mistakes: He could recall only one object after 5 minutes and could not state the name of a ballpoint pen. His clinician concluded that Rollie's **AIDS dementia** had progressed since he had last tried the MMSE just two months earlier.

Cultural Information

Questions assessing the patient's ability to name five recent presidents or five cities carry more information about education and social background than anything else; they are often irrelevant to an evaluation of medical causes of mental disorder. Less culture-bound tests include abstracting similarities and differences (How are an apple and an orange alike? What is the difference between a child and a dwarf?) Difficulty answering any of these items may suggest mental retardation, such as might occur with **homocystinuria**, Down's syndrome, or cerebral palsy.

Insight and Judgment

In the context of the mental status exam, insight refers to the patient's ideas as to what is wrong. Faulty insight may be encountered in the cognitive disorders, mental retardation, severe depression, or any of the psychoses.

Judgment refers to the patient's ability to decide what course of action is appropriate to achieve realistic goals. It is evaluated better from the assessment of the overall history than from hypothetical (and often rather silly) questions, such as how one should react to a fire that breaks out in a crowded theater. Judgment can be distorted by a variety of Axis I and Axis II mental conditions, including all causes of psychosis, delirium, and dementia.

Changes in judgment provided an early symptom of illness in several medical conditions:

- A banker with early Alzheimer's disease threw a sheaf of $5 bills out the window of his car while driving on the freeway.
- A housewife with **breast cancer** that proved metastatic to the brain flared up at her husband's boss for not promoting him to sales manager.
- A medical technician propositioned her supervisor; a subsequent medical evaluation revealed evidence of **multiple sclerosis**.

PERSONALITY CHANGE

By definition, *personality disorder* is something that is innate, present from an early age, and not caused by later-developing medical conditions. *Personality change,* on the other hand, is an alteration to a presumably already-formed personality, induced by events that occur to the individual later in life. Personality change is judged on the basis of behavior as well as more or less permanent change in mood, or affect.

Medical illnesses are prominent among the events that can induce such a change, and the condition that results is noted on

Axis I as "personality change due to [name of medical condition]." The exact nature of the patient's resulting personality characteristics would depend upon the preexisting character traits, the nature of the medical illness, and the location of the lesions it produces. Although it would seem logical that any given disease could produce just about any imaginable change in personality, in fact, a number of specific associations have been reported:

- Apathetic: **postconcussion syndrome, brain tumor** (frontal lobes), **stroke, Huntington's disease, hyperparathyroidism, adrenal insufficiency.**
- Disinhibited (inappropriately jocular or facetious): **frontal lobe tumor, stroke, Huntington's disease, syphilis, Wilson's disease.**
- Irritable: **pernicious anemia, Wilson's disease, adrenal insufficiency.**
- Obsessive–compulsive (sometimes referred to as "sticky"): **chronic fatigue syndrome, epilepsy.**
- Aggressive: **brain trauma.**
- Suspicious: **hypothyroidism.**
- Dependent: **chronic fatigue syndrome.**

Claudia Wilczynski had for many years been the receptionist for the home-state office of a U.S. senator. Claudia was valued for her ability to handle with quiet tact just about any sort of constituent, no matter how insistent or contentious. But for several months, her manner had been different—instead of directing visitors away from the Senator to seek other resources, now she seemed passively content to take names and make appointments. Her boss's appointment calendar filled up; eventually, Claudia was laid off.

While she was filling out her application for unemployment benefits, she had a seizure, right in the waiting room. A neurological workup quickly revealed a large **frontal lobe meningioma**.

Part II

60 DISORDERS

The 60 disorders that follow are by no means the only physical conditions that can cause mental disorder, but they probably account for the vast bulk of serious emotional and behavioral symptoms, the sort that cause patients and their families to consult a mental health practitioner.

Several points are important to note:

- Patients can experience far more symptoms, physical or mental, than I have detailed here. The symptoms listed in the sections that follow are generally those that occur most commonly.
- With few exceptions, most patients with these physical disorders will *not* develop mental symptoms. This creates a classical bad news–good news situation. The bad news is that because mental symptoms only occasionally are caused by physical disease, we tend to ignore the possibility of physical causes altogether. That puts us at risk for missing the occasional important, sometimes life-or-death diagnosis. The good news is obvious.
- A corollary to this is that most mental symptoms are still caused by the traditional mental disorders.

Let me make one last effort to underscore the importance of the diseases discussed. Consider the following list of the leading causes of death in the United States for 1995, as compiled by the National Center for Health Statistics:

1. Heart disease
2. Cancer
3. Stroke
4. Chronic obstructive lung disease
5. Accidents
6. Pneumonia/flu
7. Diabetes
8. AIDS
9. Suicide
10. Chronic liver disease and cirrhosis

Note that each of the first four is discussed in individual sections below, as are diabetes, AIDS, and liver failure. And infectious disease includes pneumonia and flu. In other words, much of this material is of life-and-death importance for patients, which makes it vitally important for every mental health clinician.

ADRENAL INSUFFICIENCY

Occurrence	Age of onset	Gender	Refer to
See text	Any age	Equal	Endocrinologist
What: The adrenal glands produce too little cortisone			
Physical: Weakness, fatigue, hyperpigmentation of skin, abdominal pain, fainting, nausea, vomiting, anorexia, weight loss			
Mental: Apathy, withdrawal, depression, anxiety, suicidal ideas, delirium, psychosis			

Lying across the top of each kidney, the adrenal glands look like scoops of melting ice cream. They produce hormones that promote healing and regulate salt balance in the body. Their production of these hormones is stimulated by the adrenocorticotropic hormone (ACTH), which is itself produced by the hypothalamus of the brain. This rather delicate balancing act takes place by means of a classic feedback loop: If the adrenal produces too much cortisone, the production of ACTH is shut down; too little cortisone production causes the hypothalamus to wake up and produce more ACTH.

Rarely, the adrenal gland itself is destroyed by infection or some other disease. At one time, tuberculosis was the most common culprit. Nowadays, an autoimmune disorder (the patient's immune system somehow fails to recognize portions of the patient's own body or products it makes as "self") is thought to be responsible for two-thirds or more of these cases. Adrenal insufficiency is also encountered in AIDS patients. Whatever the cause, the result is that adrenal hormone production falls dangerously, and the pituitary, stimulated by the hypothalamus, produces oceans of ACTH as it attempts to compensate. This state of affairs has long been called Addison's disease. Probably the most famous sufferer the world has ever known was John F. Kennedy, who required hormone replacement therapy throughout his presidency.

Although naturally occurring adrenal insufficiency is far from common, because adrenal steroids are often prescribed to treat a variety of diseases (infections and poison ivy, to name but two), it is not uncommon to encounter adrenal insufficiency that physicians themselves have caused.

Physical Symptoms

As the adrenal glands are eaten away by whatever disease ails them, the patient gradually develops symptoms. Perhaps most common among these is weakness, which at first may be periodic, occurring during periods of stress. It later progresses to the point of nearly complete incapacitation. Of course, the patient will also complain of fatigue, proportional to the weakness. Abdominal pain may be excruciating; other abdominal complaints, sometimes the main problem patients complain of, may include nausea, vomiting, diarrhea, loss of appetite, and weight loss. Some patients will report hypersensitivity to sounds, tastes, or smells. Low blood pressure is common; it may be manifested as fainting spells. Some patients crave salt.

The large amounts of ACTH produced by the pituitary are responsible for another characteristic symptom—hyperpigmentation. Caucasian patients develop a diffuse, bronze darkening of the skin, even affecting areas of the body not ordinarily exposed to the sun. Patients with darker skin may also note progressive deepening of skin tones. Women sometimes note reduced pubic and axillary (underarm) hair.

Sometimes tumors or other disease directly invade the hypothalamus or pituitary. Then, ACTH production is reduced, and the adrenal glands receive less stimulation than they need to produce adequate amounts of cortisone. The symptoms of the resulting adrenal insufficiency are pretty much the same as already mentioned, except that there isn't any hyperpigmentation.

Mental Symptoms

Most patients will have mental symptoms. Usually they develop gradually, often paralleling, but occasionally preceding, the onset of physical symptoms. In part because both mental and physical symptoms typically fluctuate, these patients are sometimes erroneously diagnosed as having primary mental conditions such as mood and somatoform disorders.

Personality change can be an early mental symptom. Often it is of the apathetic type, manifested by loss of interest and withdrawal from other people. In other cases, the patient may instead experience restless irritability.

Depression, which develops in up to half the patients, may be moderate or even severe. Some patients even have suicidal ideas. Mood may also be anxious or irritable. When physical and mental symptoms are at their worst—an Addisonian crisis—a classic delirium can develop with disorientation, loss of memory, and even psychosis.

Evaluation

A serum cortisol level will usually be low at 8:00 A.M.; the total amount of cortisol secreted will also be low, as determined from a collection of all the patient's urine during a 24-hour period.

Outlook

Untreated, adrenal insufficiency can be devastating and deadly, so patients should be educated to carry appropriate medical alert identification. However, steroid replacement therapy rapidly produces resolution of all symptoms, including mental symptoms. With chronic replacement therapy, a full, productive life is possible. However, even to this day, historians wrangle over the effect JFK's adrenal insufficiency might have had on the Bay of Pigs and Berlin Wall crises.

AIDS

Occurrence	Age of onset	Gender	Refer to
Frequent	Relatively young	Males predominate	Internist
What: Lethal systemic disorder caused by HIV (human immunodeficiency virus)			
Physical: Increased susceptibility to infection, numerous neurological symptoms, weakness, skin lesions			
Mental: Dementia, depression, suicidal ideas, anxiety, delirium, apathy, psychosis			

In less than two decades, AIDS has become distressingly well known. Even schoolchildren learn its usual routes of transmission: unprotected anal and vaginal intercourse, the sharing of needles by intravenous drug users, and contaminated blood products (especially a problem for patients with hemophilia). Though no one is immune, it is a disease that no one need contract. Yet it continues to infect perhaps 10 million people per year worldwide, affecting especially the young, poor minorities, and the ignorant. Currently, men outnumber women about eight to one.

Physical Symptoms

Within a few weeks of infection, over half the patients will experience an acute viral syndrome, lasting a week or two, that includes fever, sore throat, headache, aches and pains, and gastrointestinal symptoms that can include loss of appetite and weight, nausea, vomiting, and diarrhea. After these symptoms disappear, a latency period begins that can last 10 years or longer. Thereafter, stages of the disease are defined by the count of CD4+ T cells in the blood: early, above 500 cells per microliter; intermediate, from 200 to 500; advanced, below 200.

In the early phase, persistently swollen lymph nodes may appear, perhaps followed by the recurrence of an earlier, unrelated infection such as shingles or herpes. Some patients develop lesions inside the mouth. These include thrush (a cheesy, whitish exudate due to *Candida,* a fungus) and a stringy, white substance known as hairy leukoplakia, which infests the sides of the tongue. Headache can also occur as an early symptom. The blood loses its natural ability to clot, resulting in bleeding gums and an increased tendency to form bruises.

As the CD4+ T cell count plummets below 200, the body loses its ability to fight off microorganisms that a normal immune system would destroy, before they could multiply. Often, the first of these infectious agents is pneumonia (PCP) caused by *Pneumocystis carinii,* a one-celled organism that some authorities consider a protozoan, others a fungus. Patients become feverish and short of breath, and begin to cough without producing sputum ("nonproductive cough"). Virtually any other microorganism, including bacteria, fungi, syphilis, and tuberculosis, can infect the AIDS patient, causing neurological and other symptoms that the patient's compromised immune system is powerless to defend against.

Most AIDS patients will have some neurological symptoms, either in isolation or in conjunction with AIDS dementia complex (see below). They include trouble maintaining balance and walking steadily; as late manifestations, there may be incontinence of bowel or bladder. Seizures occur as a result of central nervous system (CNS) fungal infections, lymphomas, or simply in conjunction with AIDS dementia complex.

A vast array of other symptoms can appear as the disease progresses: muscle pain and weakness, skin lesions such as Kaposi's sarcoma, anemia, severe visual impairment, and chronic diarrhea.

Mental Symptoms

Mental disorders occur in the majority of all AIDS patients. Foremost among these is the AIDS dementia complex. These symptoms, which indicate that the virus has affected the CNS, don't usually appear until late in the disease. Patients may complain of difficulty concentrating, remembering, or performing complex tasks. They often become depressed or apathetic and withdrawn. In some patients, the AIDS dementia complex may be among the first symptoms to develop, even before the correct diagnosis has been made. Ultimately, around two-thirds of patients will to some degree develop this dread complication.

Other, less severely ill patients may experience apathy and a relatively mild degree of cognitive decline, including irritability, the subjective feeling of being slowed down, trouble concentrating, and minor degrees of forgetfulness. Adjustment disorders with depression or anxiety are also commonly encountered during the earlier phases of this disorder. These too-understandable psychological reactions to the fact of being ill may be difficult to differentiate from symptoms that are a biological consequence of the infection. Cause–effect issues aside, major depressive disorder affects a large number of AIDS patients. Mood disorders are likely throughout the course of AIDS: Suicidal ideas are common, and the risk of attempted or completed suicide is extremely high.

Delirium often occurs, especially when the disease progresses rapidly and the now-disoriented patient loses the ability to sustain attention and recall new information. A variety of causes for delirium is possible, including infection, disturbed metabolism, side effects of drugs, and space-occupying lesions such as tumors. At this stage, patients may become either withdrawn or vigilant and hyperactive.

Psychosis outside the syndromes of dementia and delirium is uncommon. Persecutory delusions may be attended by visual or auditory hallucinations. Manic episodes have been occasionally reported.

Evaluation

The well-known serological tests can determine whether someone has been infected with HIV, the virus responsible for AIDS.

But the only reliable laboratory indication of the extent to which the disease has progressed is the count of CD4+ T cells in the patient's blood. A falling count indicates advancing illness; a count less than 200 CD4 cells/cc is cause for prophylaxis against PCP. Because so many patients eventually become demented, all HIV-positive patients should have a screening test of cognition, such as the MMSE, for use in evaluating any future decline.

Outlook

Of course, there is still no cure, but treatment, especially with combinations of drugs, is becoming ever more hopeful. Although the best treatments available only slow the course of this disease, recent introduction of new therapeutic agents and the use of combination therapy have improved the longevity of many of these patients.

AIDS patients are far more likely to die of a secondary infection than as a direct result of the HIV agent itself. However, the rate of suicide in AIDS patients is up to 30 times more frequent than in the general population. Once symptoms of dementia appear, the outlook is grave. With advancing illness, there will be the gradual loss of self-care skills, and the patient sinks relentlessly toward dependency and merciful death.

Clinicians should also remain alert for symptoms caused by continuing drug use in patients who have contracted AIDS through drug-related activities.

ALTITUDE SICKNESS

Occurrence	Age of onset	Gender	Refer to
See text	Probably young adulthood	About equal	Anyone at sea level
What: Syndrome resulting from low blood oxygen that occurs at high altitude			
Physical: Headache, fatigue, dizziness, shortness of breath, sleepiness or insomnia			
Mental: Irritability, panic attacks, impaired judgment, delirium			

Many years ago on a commercial airliner, I responded to a request for a physician on board. My patient was a young marine, who lay in the middle of the aisle toward the rear of the plane, face up, clutching his head. During the movie, he had become acutely dizzy; when he had tried to get out of his aisle seat, he had fallen to the floor. Now, though he complained of a severe headache, he kept drifting into a doze.

With no equipment at all, I made my best effort at a physical examination. I was still puzzling over these symptoms when the captain leaned down close behind me. "The stewardess tells me he's had three beers," he murmured. I pointed out that three beers wasn't enough to account for the symptoms.

The captain coughed deferentially. "You're right, Doctor," he said. He gestured toward the marine. "But we're pressurized at 7,000 feet, and, as you know, this is just the sort of syndrome the combination of altitude and alcohol can produce."

Together we rejected an emergency landing in Indianapolis in favor of higher pressurization and a little oxygen therapy. By the time we made our scheduled landing 45 minutes later, our patient was sitting up, much improved.

Acute altitude sickness is a disorder caused by low blood-oxygen levels. Aside from frequent fliers, it affects lowlanders who stop over on high plateaus or nearly anyone who, with inadequate precautions, climbs tall mountains.

Almost by definition, permanent residents of high places, who rapidly become acclimatized to the thin atmosphere, cannot experience acute altitude sickness. (They can develop chronic altitude sickness, a different story.) It can affect nonacclimatized people at altitudes as low as 5,000 feet, and it is not at all uncommon in skiers who venture a few thousand feet higher than this in pursuit of their sport. Half or more of visitors to high altitudes (in excess of 6,000 feet) may be affected.

The risk and severity of altitude sickness are increased if there is a history of brain dysfunctioning (caused by strokes or seizures), of cardiovascular problems such as chronic obstructive lung disease, anemia, multiple heart attacks, heart failure, pneumonia, or of the use of medication or abuse of substances.

Physical Symptoms

These include headache, fatigue, dizziness, and loss of appetite. Patients become short of breath upon minor exertion, even to the extent of climbing a flight of stairs. When severe, voluntary movements may become uncoordinated. Some people experience excessive sleepiness at altitudes of only a mile or so above sea level; insomnia may be a problem for others. Seizures can also develop.

Mental Symptoms

Early symptoms may develop gradually and seem almost like an extension of the individual's normal personality quirks. These may include irritability or "feeling high."

Even at 9,000 feet, blood-oxygen saturation will be about half normal; at higher altitudes, it drops still further. Judgment becomes impaired; pilots flying without oxygen at 12,000 feet (you can *drive* that high in Colorado) report experiencing dangerous impulses, such as wanting to see how close they can get to a mountain!

With increasing anoxia, symptoms worsen. Lethargy, panic attacks, loss of memory, or disorientation may ensue. Delirium symptoms may include paranoid ideas or visual hallucinations.

Evaluation

Although blood arterial gases would be confirmatory, history and situation should make the diagnosis obvious to anyone whose judgment has not been affected by the same conditions.

Outlook

As long as the anoxia is not severe enough to cause loss of consciousness, there is little risk of permanent nervous system damage. With adequate oxygen and repressurization, symptoms will subside within a few days. Untreated and unrelieved, coma eventually yields to death.

AMYOTROPHIC LATERAL SCLEROSIS

Occurrence	Age of onset	Gender	Refer to
Uncommon	Over 40	Males predominate	Neurologist
What: Progressive deterioration of motor neurons			
Physical: Muscle weakness, cramping and fasciculations, ataxia, dysarthria, weight loss			
Mental: Reactive depression, rare dementia			

Amyotrophic lateral sclerosis (ALS) is often called Lou Gehrig's disease, after the great New York Yankee first baseman, popularly known as "The Iron Horse," whom illness forced to retire from baseball in 1939. The disease was first accurately described over 50 years earlier by Jean-Marie Charcot, the French physician even better-known for his work in describing (and, some believe, creating) grand hysteria. In ALS patients, he discovered scarring (sclerosis) in the lateral motor neuron tracts of the spinal cord. The result was, among other things, wasting of the muscles (a-myo-trophy) supplied by those nerves.

What Charcot failed to discover—the cause of this terrible affliction—remains a mystery to this day. Although some cases seem to run in families, more than 90% are sporadic. Viruses, autoimmune disorders, and environmental precipitants have been investigated, but nothing very solid has yet been discovered. No racial, ethnic, or sexual predilection has been identified in this disease, which affects around 5 people per 100,000 population. Increasing with age, this disorder typically develops in patients who are in their 40s or older.

Physical Symptoms

These are readily understood in light of the underlying pathology. Muscle wasting breeds progressive weakness of all the body's skeletal muscles, sparing only the eyes. Chewing and swallowing become difficult; the gait is disturbed. Speech becomes labored and breathing, a chore. Patients experience painful muscle cramping, especially early in the disease's course. Small bundles of muscle fibers twitch slightly, though not enough to cause gross movement of the entire body part. These movements are called fasciculations, and they are encountered in few other diseases. With loss of muscle mass, patients lose weight.

Mental Symptoms

Although the occasional patient will experience dementia, ALS usually spares the mental faculties. Depressions that occur (a not unlikely event, considering the devastation this disorder wreaks) would not be classified as "mood disorder due to ALS," because the symptoms are not directly caused by the physiological effects of the illness.

Evaluation

Electromyography (EMG) will show muscle fibrillation (persistent twitching).

Outlook

ALS patients' functional capacity will decline by about 5% per month. Although the use of respirators can keep patients alive longer today, the prognosis for useful life is little better than it was in Charcot's day.

At his farewell appearance in Yankee Stadium, Lou Gehrig said, "I consider myself the luckiest man on the face of the earth." Less than 2 years later, he was dead.

ANTIDIURETIC HORMONE, INAPPROPRIATE SECRETION

Occurrence	Age of onset	Gender	Refer to
Frequent	Especially old age	Females predominate	Endocrinologist
What: Excessive antidiuretic hormone secretion originates from physical illness or use of medication			
Physical: Headache, nausea, vomiting, blurred vision, tremor, weakness, diarrhea			
Mental: Irritability, delirium, psychosis			

Homeostasis—keeping things the same—is crucial to survival. You might almost say that until the moment of death, homeostasis is the life's work of the organism. Humans and other warm-blooded creatures especially have a seemingly endless variety of mechanisms designed to maintain constant temperature, blood chemistry, and other physiological functions. We tend to pay little attention to these systems until one of them is defeated by disease or injury. Then, physical and mental symptoms often result.

One such feedback loop is necessary to maintain the right amount of water in the body. It works through the antidiuretic hormone (ADH) that is secreted in the brain and acts on the kidneys to prevent them from excreting too much water. Without ADH, we would quickly dry up like so many prunes or raisins. But too much ADH causes otherwise normal kidneys to retain fluid when they should not, leading to dilution of the blood and reduced concentration of sodium and other serum electrolytes.

Certain physical disorders favor the development of this syndrome of inappropriate antidiuretic hormone secretion (SIADH). These include some tumors of lung, pancreas, and duodenum; other pulmonary disorders (pneumonia, tuberculosis, abscesses); and disorders of the CNS, such as encephalitis and subdural hematomas. Drugs that can stimulate ADH secretion include thiazide diuretics, phenothiazines (e.g., Thorazine), and carbamazepine (Tegretol).

Physical Symptoms

Early symptoms include headache, nausea and vomiting, blurred vision, and loss of appetite. Tremors, weakness, diarrhea, and restlessness (or sometimes lethargy) occur with continued illness. Later stages include seizures, coma, and death. Edema of the extremities, found when the body retains water due to other causes such as heart failure, is *not* a feature of the symptoms of inappropriate ADH secretion.

Mental Symptoms

Although by no means invariable, mental symptoms often occur in the course of SIADH. Least of these is irritability; cognitive disorders also occur. A delirium complicated by hallucinations or delusions may develop.

Evaluation

The serum sodium level is low. It will be especially notable if it drops precipitously through the course of a single day, as the patient takes on a heavy water load. Urine will be abnormally concentrated.

Outlook

Excessive water drinking can be notoriously difficult to prevent, especially if the patient hides the behavior. Some authors suggest that more than 10% of *all* schizophrenia patients drink themselves to death as a result of SIADH. But if the patient is able to curtail drinking behavior, the symptoms are rapidly self-correcting. Of course, in some cases, ultimate outcome may be determined by an underlying physical disease such as lung cancer or encephalitis.

Special Note on Primary Polydypsia

Some mental patients, notably those with long-standing schizophrenia, drink excessive amounts of fluid (polydypsia). Sometimes they do this in response to delusions or hallucinations.

Although the behavior may be obvious, some patients conceal their excessive drinking. Normally, even very high water loads will simply be excreted by the kidneys, with little harm done. But when a patient secretes abnormal amounts of ADH and drinks excessive fluids, symptoms of water toxicity occur, as described earlier. Best estimates suggest that this disorder afflicts around 10% of schizophrenia patients, in the vast majority of whom excessive water drinking is never suspected.

BRAIN ABSCESS

Occurrence	Age of onset	Gender	Refer to
Uncommon	Peaks in 30s	Males predominate	Neurologist
What: Brain infection leaves behind space-occupying lesion			
Physical: Headache, fever, seizures, nausea, vomiting, stiff neck, focal neurological symptoms			
Mental: Lethargy, range of cognitive symptoms			

An abscess is just a pocket of pus. Depending upon its exact location, a brain abscess can have a variety of effects, some of them extremely serious, upon behavior and thought. Because abscesses can be generated by so many organisms, the cause can be as varied as the symptoms.

As serious—often deadly—as the symptoms can be, a brain abscess poses far less threat now that it did 50 years ago. There are two reasons for this.

1. With CT scan and MRI, it is now far easier to diagnose the fact and extent of brain abscess.
2. Antibiotics effective against a wide spectrum of microorganisms have made treatment much more practical.

As you might imagine, however, in Third World countries, brain abscess remains relatively common. Men predominate by about two to one.

How does infection get started in an organ that resides in a tightly sealed box and is remarkably resistant to infection? Of course, any neurosurgical procedure carries with it some risk of infection, but only a tiny percent of brain abscesses are generated by such a lawyer's delight. In about one-fourth of the cases, the infection is carried to the brain from some other part of the body. The most common cause is by extension from some adjacent structure in the skull—an infected sinus or ear, for example. Infected teeth are responsible for about 10% of cases, another good reason to brush daily. Other health problems that render brain abscess more likely include AIDS and snorting cocaine.

Physical Symptoms

Brain abscess begins relatively rapidly and usually runs its course within a couple of weeks. The symptoms are those of any expanding mass lesion in the brain. Of course, they will depend upon the site of the abscess; frontal is most likely, occipital least. About half the patients will have fever, and two-thirds or more will have headache. A large minority will have seizures, and if pressure builds up inside the skull, nausea, vomiting, and stiff neck will develop. Focal neurological symptoms include hemiplegia (paralysis of one side of the body), blindness on one side of the visual field (hemianopsia), aphasia and anomia, paralysis of facial muscles and of the muscles that move the eyeball. Speech problems may be apparent. Patients with an abscess in the cerebellum (at the base of the skull) may have tremor, trouble walking, and nystagmus.

Mental Symptoms

Most patients will experience some change in cognitive status. This may be confined to disorientation and lethargy, especially likely when the abscess is in the frontal lobes, but all gradations of alertness, even to frank coma, have been observed.

Evaluation

As noted above, CT scan and MRI are the standard.

Outlook

For the first half of this century, mortality rate approximated 50%. With modern diagnosis and treatment, it has fallen to around 10%. Even so, up to half the survivors will have some kind of residual neurological deficit.

BRAIN TUMOR

Occurrence	Age of onset	Gender	Refer to
Frequent	Any age	Slight female excess	Neurologist
What: Tissue growth in brain displaces normal structures			
Physical: Headache, vomiting, dizziness, seizures, focal neurological symptoms			
Mental: Loss of memory, cognitive decline, dementia, personality change (apathy, disinhibition), depression, dissociation, psychosis			

Brain tumors* affect a lot of patients, causing nearly 100,000 deaths per year in this country. Even so, they still are not exactly commonplace.

They can be categorized in several ways, but what matters most to the person who has one is this: What is the likelihood of my disability or death? The answer depends not only on the type of tumor (malignant or benign), but also on its location, for a "benign" tumor growing relentlessly at a place in the brain where it cannot be treated may have a very poor prognosis indeed.

Most brain tumors actually don't start there at all but are metastatic from somewhere else in the body. Lung cancer (in men) and breast cancer (in women) are the ones most likely to take up residence in the brain, though many other primary cancers can do the same.

---

*Properly speaking, we are discussing intracranial tumors, some of which are tumors of the brain itself. Others, such as meningiomas, are tumors of the coverings of the brain, blood vessels, and other structures. All can produce mental symptoms.

Physical Symptoms

The symptoms a tumor will cause are mainly determined by the location within the brain and its growth rate, though the type of tumor may have some effect, too. Metastatic cancers are more likely to appear and evolve rapidly (days or weeks).

However, most tumors have certain symptoms in common. Headache is the first symptom in about half the patients. It may occur at night, or be present upon first awakening, and is usually experienced on the side of the head where the tumor is located. Once pressure begins to build up inside the skull, dizziness or vomiting may occur, sometimes without the usual warning symptom of nausea. Increasing pressure within the skull will eventually lead to a dilated pupil ("blown pupil") on the same side as the tumor, an ominous sign. Seizures occur in around half of all patients.

Metastatic tumors tend to evolve rapidly and are associated with seizures and worsening headache. Other ("focal") neurological symptoms include gait disturbance, hearing loss, double or blurred vision, speech or language problems, and a host of muscle weaknesses and paralyses that are determined by the extent and exact location of the tumor. With continued enlargement may come loss of control of bowels or bladder.

Mental Symptoms

As you might imagine, progressive cognitive decline is a characteristic feature. The patient gradually thinks less quickly. With further progression occur the typical symptoms of dementia, including aphasia, apraxia, amnesia, and loss of memory and executive functioning.

Especially found in frontal lobe tumors, two types of personality change have been noted. Apathetic personality change (not a personality *disorder*, which would imply pathology that persists from the time of adolescence throughout adult life) suggests loss of spontaneous action and a lack of appropriate concern. In disinhibited personality change, the patient's behavior may become impulsive, perhaps to the point of violence or rudeness, or some other form of social offense. Interviews with relatives or others who know the patient well may be necessary to determine the extent to which behavior has altered.

Both depression and mania have been reported, though depression is by far the more common. Moods may shift rapidly; sleep, appetite, and sexual functioning may alter, even without much in the way of an apparent mood disorder.

Some patients experience dissociative symptoms such as derealization, depersonalization, or *déjà vu* (the sensation of thinking you have previously experienced a location or situation, when this is probably not the case). Hallucinations can also occur; their type (usually visual or olfactory, though auditory hallucinations have been reported) will depend on the location of the tumor. Persecutory delusions are sometimes encountered in temporal lobe tumors. Capgras delusions have been particularly associated with brain tumors. These patients become persuaded that their relatives have been replaced by exact doubles; that is, although the person in question looks just like a relative, the patient "knows" that the person is really an imposter, or perhaps an alien that has taken over the body of a loved one.

Evaluation

Short of brain biopsy, CT scan or MRI will usually provide the most reliable diagnosis.

Outlook

A benign tumor (such as a meningioma), located where it can be surgically removed, is fully compatible with a normal life span. Unhappily, metastatic and malignant primary tumors are more common by far. Then, life span is often measured in months.

CANCER

Occurrence	Age of onset	Gender	Refer to
Common	Increases with age	See text	Oncologist
What: Tissue growth out of control somewhere in the body			
Physical: Varies with site, weakness, pain, anorexia, malaise			
Mental: Depression, anxiety, suicidal ideas, delirium, posttraumatic stress disorder (PTSD)			

Cancer. The very sound of the word terrifies. We avoid it whenever we can. We use euphemisms such as "tumor," "mass," or "growth." Persons born during the last week of June or the first three weeks of July scramble for alternative names ("Moon Child") for their astrological sign. Small wonder, you might think, that more cancer* patients don't have emotional problems.

As it happens, nearly half do. Often this is some form of a mood disorder, either a major depressive episode or an adjustment disorder with depressed mood. A variety of factors predict reactive mental symptoms in cancer patients:

- A previous history of mental illness, such as mood disorder or alcoholism.
- More serious cancer symptoms (disability, malnutrition, intense pain).
- Type of treatment (side effects of chemotherapy, disfiguring surgery, such as breast removal, or surgery affecting the head and neck).
- Inadequate support system, including absent family, few friends, inadequate education from healthcare professionals.
- In some cancers, offering a treatment choice may diminish the likelihood of emotional distress.

---

*Carcinoma, or cancer, technically refers only to malignant tumors arising from epithelial (skin) cells; it affects skin and the lining of internal organs. Malignancies that affect muscle, cartilage, and bone arise from connective tissue and are properly called sarcomas.

- Mental morbidity does *not* seem to be associated with the patient's age, sex, marital or socioeconomic status.

Usually, mental symptoms are less likely in patients who have not yet been told that they have cancer, suggesting the self-evident conclusion that some mental symptoms are reactive to the emotional blow this diagnosis inflicts. Only a few cancers outside the CNS appear to cause mental symptoms in some direct, physiological way, not just as a reaction to the knowledge of illness. One is carcinoid, discussed elsewhere in this volume. Multiple myeloma and certain lung tumors also secrete hormones that can affect the emotions. However, up to 50% of patients with cancer of the pancreas report depressive symptoms even before the physical symptoms appear. It seems entirely possible that with this tumor, some apparently unique biological process directly affects mood.

Two other angles on the relation between mental disorder and cancer seem important to note here.

1. Although it has been often stated that depression may itself constitute a risk factor for cancer, recent epidemiological studies provide little support for such an idea.
2. On a brighter note, recent well-designed studies find that supportive emotional therapy for patients with a variety of cancers may not only improve the quality of life, but even help prolong it.

Of course, the sexual predilection for cancer will depend on its type (lung cancers occur largely in men, breast cancers in women). But, whereas non-cancer-related mood disorders are about twice as likely to occur in women, there is no such gender bias among cancer patients.

Physical Symptoms

These will depend largely upon the site of the cancer and may change as it spreads. By local enlargement or invasion, cancer can encroach upon normal functioning anywhere in the body, interfering with breathing, digestion, elimination, sexual ability, strength, and motor and sensory nerve functioning. Symptoms common to many cancers include weakness, loss of appetite and weight, pain, and malaise (feeling sick).

Mental Symptoms

As noted, these are most likely to be depressive in nature. Cancer patients can have a full range of mood symptoms, though mania is hardly ever encountered, no surprise. Often, depression seems reactive to the news or secondary to the fact of chronic illness, but severe major depressive episodes with melancholia may also develop. Cancer patients commit suicide at a rate higher than the general population.

Anxiety symptoms are nearly as frequent as depression, especially early in the diagnostic process, when the patient is suspicious, but not yet certain, of bad news. Panic attacks and other anxiety symptoms may also occur in patients who are experiencing pain or whose air exchange is compromised by lung cancer. Nearly one-fourth of cancer patients may suffer from delirium brought on by drug treatment, malnutrition, or as a terminal event. And some patients, experiencing disfigurement or the loss of a body part (breast cancer is the classical example), may experience symptoms that allow a DSM-IV diagnosis of PTSD.

Evaluation

In many cases, definitive diagnosis can be made only by biopsy. But a variety of radiological and biochemical tests may help confirm suspicions raised by history and physical examination.

Outlook

No general statement is possible. In some cases, surgery, radiation therapy, or chemotherapy can offer outright cure. Other patients may live only a few weeks beyond initial diagnosis. The individual's place on this spectrum is defined by general health, site and type of cancer, and the stage at which it was detected.

CARCINOID SYNDROME

Occurrence	Age of onset	Gender	Refer to
Frequent	Any age	About equal	Endocrinologist
What: Intestinal tumors (among others) secrete serotonin and other hormones			
Physical: Diarrhea, symptoms of local growth of tumor			
Mental: Flushing of face and entire body			

The number of disorders that present with only *one* mental health symptom is small, and carcinoid tumor is it. Carcinoid tumors got their name because early pathologists thought that, with their regular appearance and slow growth, they only *looked* like cancer. But they're malignant, right enough, dangerous enough to kill. Yet who outside the medical professions have ever heard of them?

These tumors largely originate in the intestines and metastasize to the liver. Once there, a small percentage of them cause the peculiar symptom of flushing. Of course, flushing (or blushing) can have quite a number of causes, not the least of which is embarrassment or concern that people are watching (think social phobia, for one). But in carcinoid syndrome, the growth of endocrine tissue at odd places throughout the body causes symptoms. These tumors can occur at nearly any age, from the teens onward, but peak in the 40s and 50s.

Physical Symptoms

Common symptoms include bleeding into the intestine (producing dark, blood-containing stool called melena), abdominal pain, and sometimes obstruction of the flow of food through the intestines. One of the most common places for them to occur is in the appendix, in which case there may be no symptoms at all. When they secrete hormones, as they sometimes do, carcinoid tumors can cause diarrhea and heart disease (rarely, right heart failure). Loss of blood pressure may also be noted during attacks. Sometimes constriction of the bronchi in the lungs produces wheezing similar to an asthma attack.

Mental Symptom

Note the singular, "symptom." Early in the course of this illness, flushing may be initiated by stress. Eating food or drinking alcohol can also cause flushing in these patients. It isn't just the face and neck that can be affected; patients may flush all over their bodies. Facial flushing is occasionally so severe that small blood vessels of the face become permanently dilated as a result. Of course, flushing is also seen in a number of other disorders, including menopause, pheochromocytoma (q.v.), and alcohol use. I've included flushing as a mental symptom, because it is such a prominent symptom of social phobia.

Evaluation

Most patients will have high blood levels of the breakdown products of serotonin. These can be quantified in 24-hour urine samples.

Outlook

By the time patients develop the symptoms of carcinoid syndrome, they usually have metastatic disease. As a result, most people live only 2–3 years after first beginning to blush. For patients identified early, surgery can be curative.

CARDIAC ARRHYTHMIAS

Occurrence	Age of onset	Gender	Refer to
Common	Any age	See text	Cardiologist
What: Heartbeat that is faster, slower, or less regular than normal			
Physical: Palpitations, faintness, dizziness, fatigue			
Mental: Anxiety, delirium			

Until you fall in love, you mostly aren't aware of your heart. It was designed to go unnoticed, in which it largely succeeds, so long as it beats steadily and slowly. Cardiac arrhythmias produce the sensation of palpitation, which, though not quite so universal an experience as sneezing, is extremely common nonetheless.

The heartbeat is controlled by electrical impulses that arise within the heart itself. Most of the events that we call palpitations—heartbeats that are faster, slower, or less regular than normal—are caused by abnormalities in the way these electrical impulses are generated or conducted throughout the heart muscle. There are two basic types of abnormality of heartbeat: disorders of rate, and disorders of rhythm.

Disorders of rhythm are caused by extrasystolic heartbeats. These are individual beats that occur at a time different from what would be indicated by the normal, steady beat of the heart. They are often followed by a pause that can produce the alarming sensation that the heart has stopped completely. Most normal adults have extrasystolic beats every day and simply do not realize it. Of course, irregular heartbeat can also indicate pathology.

As you might imagine, disorders of rate include "too fast" and "too slow." Too fast (tachycardia) occurs when something other than exercise raises the heartbeat above its normal rate of around 60–100 beats per minute (individuals vary considerably in resting heart rate). Most tachycardias are caused by abnormalities of the heart's own electrical firing mechanism, but some are caused by disease that lies outside the heart itself. Disorders that can drive up heart rate include fever, anemia, and hyperthyroidism. Too slow (bradycardia) is usually due to something that impedes conduction of the firing impulse from one part of the heart to another. However, athletes who have trained hard and some older people may have heart rates as slow as 50 beats per minute and still be normal.

It is hard to make a general statement about gender and cardiac arrhythmias. Women tend to have some of the less threatening, though still alarming conditions such as paroxysmal atrial tachycardia. Men suffer the bulk of serious heart disease, and therefore are more likely to have the abnormality of heartbeat that demands medical attention.

Physical Symptoms

Patients use a great many terms to express the sensation of palpitation. Tachycardias may be experienced as the heart "working like a piston" or "running away with itself." They may begin and end either gradually or, in certain types, with the suddenness of an electrical switch being thrown. Extrasystoles, if noted at all, will feel like a "hard thumping," "pounding," "fluttering," or "skipping."

If the disorder of heartbeat is serious, circulation may slow down. The resulting lack of oxygen (hypoxia) may produce only a sensation of faintness or dizziness, sometimes expressed as feeling lightheaded. Fatigue may also present a problem. However, symptoms of heart failure can develop in especially severe cases.

Mental Symptoms

Patients with heartbeat problems commonly experience anxiety, due either to low blood oxygen or to the fear that accompanies the perception of a faltering heart. Anxiety is often experienced especially at night, when patients can typically devote more time to worry. (The reverse relationship should also be noted: Along with other somatic symptoms, panic attacks commonly provoke palpitations.)

Adolescence is the time people begin to become aware of imperfections of their anatomy and physiology. When reassured that palpitations are normal, most young people will learn to regard these experiences as, at worst, an inconvenience. Less sophisticated or more insecure patients may regard their palpitations as portending doom. Then, anxiety or somatoform disorders may ensue.

Occasionally, patients with a form of bradycardia called sick sinus syndrome (the sinus node is the heart's normal, internal pacemaker) will develop a delirium from too little blood flow to the brain.

Evaluation

Electrocardiogram.

Outlook

In most cases, those palpitations that are not benign can be stabilized with medication.

CEREBROVASCULAR ACCIDENT

Occurrence	Age of onset	Gender	Refer to
Common	Increases with age	Slight excess of males	Neurologist
What: Death of brain tissue due to blockage of artery			
Physical: Focal neurological symptoms, agnosia, amnesia, aphasia, apraxia			
Mental: Various cognitive disorders, personality change, depression, mania, psychosis			

When in 1913 Woodrow Wilson became the 28th President of the United States, he already had had several warnings of the disease that incapacitated him during much of his second term in office and would eventually kill him. High blood pressure from his young adult years had probably contributed to an episode of near blindness in his left eye in 1906. He suffered intensely from severe headaches while serving as president. At least two previous, smaller episodes of the same disease may have caused him to become somewhat impulsive, sensitive, and arbitrary.

This disorder, cerebrovascular accident (CVA), is commonly referred to as stroke. It is a common disorder, affecting about 150 persons per 100,000 general population each year. It is more common in Black than in White patients, and slightly more common in men than in women. Although stroke can occur at any age, the likelihood increases dramatically with advancing age; people between the ages of 60 and 80 are especially vulnerable. Risk is increased by hypertension, heart disease, and diabetes.

There are three principal types of stroke:

- Thrombotic, in which a blood clot forms in a vessel in the brain.
- Embolic, in which an obstruction (e.g., it could be a blood clot or a bit of fat) formed elsewhere in the body travels to the brain and lodges there
- Hemorrhagic, in which there is bleeding into the substance of the brain.

The end result in each case is that brain tissue, deprived of its blood and oxygen supplies, dies (death of an organ due to anoxia is called infarction).

In September 1919, in the midst of trying to persuade the Senate to ratify the creation of his beloved League of Nations, Wilson suffered a massively debilitating stroke that for the next 7 months left him unable even to meet with his cabinet. When once again alert enough to attempt useful work, the President of the United States could no longer concentrate well enough to follow the thread of any idea that had not been presented to him before he fell ill. Unaware of the degree of his infirmity, Wilson was in fact demented, a fact his wife and closest advisors conspired to withhold from the country for the last year and a half of his presidency. One victim was the League, which never did receive the Senate's endorsement.

Physical Symptoms

These can vary widely, depending on the exact location of the infarct. Of course, a massive lesion in an area of the brain that controls motor functioning will produce the (usually) sudden onset of catastrophic defects that are all too obvious. These include paralysis, spasticity, change in posture, incontinence, loss of sensation, partial blindness, and even mutism. Other neurological symptoms may become apparent only upon closer observation:

- *Agnosia.* The patient cannot recognize familiar people, shapes, or objects, or may not be able to state their use.

- *Amnesia.* The patient cannot recall recent information or retain new information.
- *Aphasia.* The use of language suffers through trouble speaking or loss of speech comprehension.
- *Apraxia.* Patients cannot do on command that which they are able to do spontaneously (such as kicking a ball). Patients with constructional apraxia have difficulty copying designs.
- *Executive functioning.* This means that the patient has difficulty following a sequence of directions or tasks, such as dressing.
- *Neglect and denial.* There may be neglect of grooming on the affected side (e.g., hair brushing only on the left) or denial that there is anything much the matter.

Mental Symptoms

Although most patients remain conscious, a variety of mental syndromes can be produced by stroke. Of course, all variations of cognitive disorder can occur, especially dementia.

Personality Change

Most notably occurring when frontal lobes are damaged, patients might become apathetic, euphoric, facetious, disinhibited, jocular, or impulsive. Perhaps the apparent loss of judgment suffered by Woodrow Wilson in the months preceding his catastrophic 1919 stroke was an example of such a personality change.

Depression

Around one-fourth of stroke patients suffer from depressed mood, failing interests or concentration, change in appetite and sleep, fatigue, guilt, and suicidal ideas. They may at times have enough of these symptoms to warrant a diagnosis of major depressive disorder. Depression may sometimes be inappropriately diagnosed in a patient who does not feel depressed but looks it because of emotional incontinence. Unrelated to current mood, such patients may become instantly tearful without adequate provocation, and so appear to have sudden, wide swings of mood. (Less frequently, these patients may become suddenly giddy or laugh.) Concomitant anxiety symptoms are not the rule, though they may be present.

Mania

Bipolar mood disorder may be suggested in some patients who develop mania-like symptoms: grandiosity, reduced need for sleep, talkativeness, flight of ideas, easy distractibility, increased activity levels, poor judgment. These patients may deny or downplay their obvious neurological deficits. Manic symptoms may resolve, recur, or persist.

Psychosis

The visual hallucination is the principal psychotic symptom associated with stroke, or with any other neurological disorder, for that matter. These patients may see only shapes, but sometimes they may discern the formed images of people or scenes. Eye-blinking may cause the images to change. Auditory hallucinations rarely occur in vascular disease. When delusions occur, they are often persecutory.

Evaluation

CT scan or MRI can provide definitive visualization of the site and extent of damage.

Outlook

As you might imagine, prognosis varies tremendously, based on a number of factors. Site and extent of the lesion are paramount, but the patient's age is also very important: Because of the greater plasticity of the developing brain, children are much more likely than adults to recover fully or partially.

Special Note on Transient Ischemic Attacks (TIAs)

These are symptoms caused by anoxia too brief to produce brain tissue death (ischemia means "reduced blood supply due to a narrowed artery"). By definition, TIAs last less than 24 hours, but they may herald the eventual development of a completed stroke in the same region of the brain. They can be identified by headache, numbness, dizziness, and many other neurological symptoms. Trouble speaking, amnesia, and changes in behavior also may be noted, but all revert to normal within a few hours. The development of TIA should be cause for great concern and immediate referral to a neurologist.

CHRONIC OBSTRUCTIVE LUNG DISEASE

Occurrence	Age of onset	Gender	Refer to
Common	40s to 60s	Males predominate	Internist
What: Loss of elasticity and absorptive surface area of the lung			
Physical: Shortness of breath, cough, dusky skin hue, headache, tremor			
Mental: Anxiety, panic attacks, depression, insomnia, delirium, dementia			

This collection of diseases is as lethal and commonplace as any on earth. Together, the ordinary pulmonary disorders of asthma, bronchitis, and emphysema affect nearly half the world's population, though far fewer than that number ever have important symptoms. In the 21st century, with the marketing of cigarettes continuing unabated throughout Third World countries, the situation will probably only worsen. Currently, in our own country, far more men are affected, though women are increasingly puffing their way to a strong second-place finish.

Chronic obstructive lung disease (its acronym, COLD, is a bitter gibe) comprises two principal disorders: chronic bronchitis and emphysema. The former refers to the increased production of mucus in the upper respiratory tract that persists for several months each year. The latter is even more serious—with it, there is actual loss of lung surface area, across which gases must diffuse from air to blood and back again. In both conditions, there is a narrowing of the air passages and a loss of lung elasticity; the patient has to work hard just to draw, and release, each breath.

After smoking (and secondhand smoke), principal causes include air pollution, infection, and occupation hazards (think asbestosis and miner's lung). The incidence begins to increase when patients are in their 40s and 50s.

Physical Symptoms

Bronchitis patients have a persistent cough that produces sputum. Because they don't get quite enough oxygen to their peripheral tissues, many have skin of a dusky hue (cyanosis). As long as they are resting, those with only moderate disease may not experience much physical distress, other than fatigue. With more severe disease, they may develop right heart failure.

Emphysema patients typically have shortness of breath (dyspnea) when they exert themselves even minimally. They cough less and produce less sputum than do bronchitis patients. They tend to weigh less than they should and find it hard work to breathe, even when resting. A severely affected patient will use the accessory muscles of respiration to help with the effort of breathing. Sitting forward in a chair, such a patient strains with chest and arm muscles to force air out. (We ordinarily breathe in using only the diaphragm; exhaling is accomplished by gravity and the normal elasticity of chest and lungs.) Because they find it so hard to get air *out* of the lungs, some COLD patients will breathe out through pursed lips, perhaps grunting at the beginning of expiration. After years of this effort, the chest becomes barrel-shaped. Cyanosis of the extremities is not usually present.

Not only do COLD patients have difficulty getting oxygen into the system, but it is also a struggle to get carbon dioxide out. The combination of hypoxia and excessive blood carbon dioxide (hypercapnia) yields an intense ache at the front or back of the head that can last for hours, a rapid tremor of the extremities, and sometimes a jerking of muscle groups.

Mental Symptoms

Picture yourself deep underwater, trying to breathe without an oxygen tank. This is the way COLD patients feel much of the time. Suffocation is intensely anxiety provoking; these patients may become agitated and have many symptoms of panic attack (though the appropriate diagnosis, in most cases, would be anxiety disorder due to COLD). As the patient approaches end-stage disease, this sensation may intensify. The fear of sudden death is, of course, quite realistic. Agitation and insomnia are frequent accompaniments.

Depression is also common, with loss of interest in former activities and even fleeting thoughts of suicide. Sexual ability and even interest often fall prey to anxiety, depression, and the effects of multiple medications.

As blood oxygen decreases and carbon dioxide increases, delirium may develop. Attention wanders, judgment deteriorates, and apathy and drowsiness set in. After several periods of respiratory crisis, dementia may lead to impaired memory and abstract reasoning; psychotic symptoms such as visual hallucinations may occur. Any of these manifestations of severe cognitive disorder may worsen with periods of reduced sensory stimulation ("sundowning").

Evaluation

Pulmonary function studies (respirometry) will measure the compromise of the patient's breathing capacity. Blood-gas determinations will help evaluate the effects of such incapacity.

Outcome

Around one-fourth of even severely ill COLD patients will survive 5 years or longer. The quality of life may be improved with the use of nasal oxygen and, seemingly paradoxically, exercise. Regardless of stage of disease, patients who are able to conquer their addiction to nicotine will at least slow the progression of their disease.

CONGESTIVE HEART FAILURE

Occurrence	Age of onset	Gender	Refer to
Common	Increases with age	Males predominate	Cardiologist
What: Heart disease or arrhythmia causes the heart to lose pumping efficiency			
Physical: Shortness of breath, weakness, fatigue, edema, cyanosis, cold extremities			
Mental: Anxiety, panic attacks, depression, insomnia, delirium			

Heart failure is the inability to pump enough blood to nourish all the tissues of the body. Of course, it isn't a *complete* failure, only a relative inability. When the heart truly fails, the patient dies. On a cardiologist's report card, "Failure" really means that the heart earns a C-minus or a D.

Failure occurs when the heart becomes too weak to cope with the load placed upon it. Often this happens because a myocardial infarction (heart attack) weakens, or even kills, part of the heart muscle. Another common cause is a cardiac arrhythmia that reduces the heart's efficiency, throwing it into failure. Hyperthyroidism in a pregnant woman, anemia, and infection are unrelated medical conditions that can precipitate failure in an already weakened heart.

Physical Symptoms

Shortness of breath (dyspnea—literally, "difficult breathing") is an early symptom of heart failure. It occurs when the left side of the heart, which receives blood from the lungs and pumps it out to the body, cannot do its job effectively and fluid backs up in the lungs. At first, exertion may only make the patient pant and puff more that usual. (Of course, everyone becomes short of breath with enough exertion—the difference is in degree.) As the failure worsens, the patient tolerates exercise less and less well, until even climbing a few stairs may become too taxing. Eventually, just lying flat in bed becomes impossible: The patient wheezes, breathing in rapid, shallow gasps. To allow as much fluid as possible to drain away from the lungs, the patient may even sleep sitting up (a condition known as orthopnea—clinicians sometimes pseudoquantify it by speaking of "three-pillow orthopnea"). When patients who must sleep propped up roll off their pillows, they may awaken with coughing and acute shortness of breath, called paroxysmal nocturnal dyspnea.

The right side of the heart receives blood from the body and pumps it out to the lungs for oxygenation; when there is failure of the right side, fluid backs up in the body, and the extremities, especially the legs and ankles, become swollen with edema. Of course, both sides may fail together, producing a mixture of symptoms.

Heart failure also causes weakness and fatigue. Because the transfer of gases in the lungs is impeded, a patient may have blueness of nails, lips, or extremities (cyanosis). Decreasing circulation causes feet and fingers to feel cold, both to the touch and to the patient. Blood pooling in the extremities causes edema that is especially noticeable in the ankles and the shins; it is usually worst in the evenings. Impotence may occur. Severe heart failure may be associated with nausea, vomiting, loss of appetite, and, ultimately, weight loss. Jaundice may be a late symptom.

Mental Symptoms

Anxiety symptoms, including panic attacks, are common in patients with heart failure. Anxiety is especially likely when the patient awakens at night, unable to breathe. Then, sitting up on the edge of the bed will usually relieve both the dyspnea and the anxiety.

The depression that commonly affects heart failure patients may simply be a reaction to feeling sick; often it is *not* associated with features of melancholia such as guilt feelings and loss of appetite and weight. However, even patients with moderate congestive heart failure commonly complain of insomnia, and more severely ill patients may lose the will to live.

With severe heart failure, oxygen saturation of the blood declines, and the amount of blood pumped to vital organs is also reduced. As a result, the brain becomes oxygen-starved and cognitive symptoms develop. Patients may complain of feeling confused or being drowsy; a delirium, possibly with psychosis, may ensue.

Evaluation

Chest X-ray and echocardiogram will reveal changes in heart size typical of failure. Serial mental status exams (such as the MMSE) can be used to evaluate the progress of cognitive disorder.

Outlook

Although excellent treatment to strengthen heartbeat and eliminate excess fluid from the body is available, many patients die suddenly, without warning. Prognosis is improved when there is a definitive correction available for a precipitating factor such as hyperthyroidism, pregnancy, or a defective heart valve.

CRYPTOCOCCOSIS

Occurrence	Age of onset	Gender	Refer to
Frequent	Especially young adulthood	Males exceed females	Internist
What: A fungus transmitted in pigeon droppings, especially affecting AIDS patients			
Physical: Headache, stiff neck, fever, nausea, blurred vision, staggering gait, focal symptoms			
Mental: Irritability, disorientation, dementia, mania, psychosis			

Off and on for more than 50 years, San Francisco newspaper columnist Herb Caen railed against pigeons, much to the indignation of Bay Area bird fanciers. Caen's hatred of pigeons had to do more with esthetics than with illness, and indeed, the number of illnesses humans contract from birds is small (don't count indigestion from too much holiday turkey). In fact, fungal infections might escape our attention altogether, were it not that AIDS patients are so vulnerable to such infections. However, cryptococcosis has long been associated with other chronic, debilitating conditions, including leukemia, Hodgkin's disease, tuberculosis, diabetes mellitus, and systemic lupus erythematosus.

In the 1990s, 80% or more of cryptococcosis patients had AIDS, and 5–10% of AIDS patients developed cryptococcosis. Overall, men outnumber women by two to one.

Physical Symptoms

When first diagnosed, most patients have symptoms of meningitis, most often headache; when present, stiff neck and fever tend to be relatively mild. Other symptoms include nausea, blurring of vision, and a staggering gait. Seizures may also be present. A cystic abscess of the brain (q.v.) may develop, as may granuloma, which is a group of cells that gather anywhere in the body to fight infection. Abscesses and granulomas can become quite large and induce focal neurological symptoms.

Mental Symptoms

Irritability, disorientation and, eventually, dementia constitute the predominant mental symptoms. However, the occasional patient has presented with mania or psychosis.

Evaluation

Viewing cerebrospinal fluid that has been bathed in India ink will reveal the typical, encapsulated appearance of this yeast. Here, for once, the diagnostic gold standard has not changed for generations!

Outlook

Untreated, nearly all cryptococcosis patients die. But treatment with new antibiotics cures around two-thirds of patients who do not have AIDS.

CUSHING'S SYNDROME

Occurrence	Age of onset	Gender	Refer to
Frequent	Young adulthood	Females predominate	Endocrinologist
What: Adrenal gland overactivity (or prescribed adrenal steroid medication) causes excess cortisone production			
Physical: Truncal obesity, moon face, "buffalo hump," weakness, increased body hair, oily skin			
Mental: Depression, anxiety, delirium, psychosis			

Cushing's syndrome is an endocrine disorder that was named for a surgeon, which may be the only time that has happened. It happened because Harvey Cushing, a neurosurgeon who practiced at Johns Hopkins, Harvard, and Yale Universities during the early 20th century, operated on a number of patients whose pituitary tumors caused them quite a bit of mischief.

The pituitary gland is the so-called master endocrine gland, located on the under side of the brain. It regulates the secretions of many of the body's endocrine functions. This includes telling the adrenal glands how much cortisone to produce. Whereas a little cortisone is a fine thing—among other actions, it promotes healing of injured tissues—too much of the stuff creates havoc with the patient's physical and mental well-being.

As you might imagine, a pituitary tumor is not the only opportunity one has to develop Cushing's syndrome. Primary tumors (about half are malignant) of the adrenal glands and a few other causes can provoke the symptoms, too. But the most common cause of Cushing-type symptoms comes from physicians prescribing steroids as treatment for a variety of disorders. Each year, Cushing's syndrome will affect as many as 10 of every 1 million adults.

Physical Symptoms

Patients gain weight in a pattern that is both distinctive and somewhat peculiar. There is obesity of the torso but not the arms and legs; a fat pad develops across the back of the neck, where it joins the shoulders, creating a "buffalo hump" appearance. The face also rounds out so that the patient appears "moon-faced." (Because the face also becomes ruddy, "Mars-faced" might be a more accurate description). There is muscle wasting, especially of the large muscles of the thighs and upper arms, with corresponding weakness. Blood pressure rises. Women may develop signs of virilization: increased body or facial hair, scant or absent menses. Men can become impotent. The skin sometimes is oily, and acne may ensue.

Mental Symptoms

These are even more varied than the physical symptoms, and half or more of Cushing patients have them. Most common is a depressive syndrome whose symptoms look just like major depressive disorder: low mood, crying spells, tiredness, interval or terminal sleep disturbance, irritability, poor concentration and loss of memory, suicidal ideas, and either agitation or psychomotor retardation. Anxiety symptoms may be prominent, and some patients may have cognitive problems that resemble a dementia or delirium.

Within the first 4–5 days of starting or increasing steroid medication, euphoria and sleep loss suggestive of a manic episode may develop; most patients then progress to depressive symptoms. Hallucinations (especially visual) may also occur during a steroid psychosis; paranoid ideas may also occur, but they are reportedly rare.

Evaluation

A history of recent use of steroid-containing mediation will usually suggest the diagnosis. An elevated total corticosteroid content of a 24-hour urine specimen will confirm a diagnosis of Cushing's syndrome due to other causes.

Outcome

Mental symptoms usually abate completely once the underlying cause has been addressed. Happily, surgical techniques have improved since the days of Harvey Cushing, and most patients can look forward to a normal life span.

DEAFNESS

Occurrence	Age of onset	Gender	Refer to
Common	Bimodal	About equal	Audiologist
What: Reduced hearing acuity			
Physical: Impaired hearing			
Mental: Paranoid ideas			

It was in the early part of the 20th century (1915, in fact) that Emil Kraepelin first suggested a link between deafness and mental illness. He called it "paranoia of the deaf," a term that has not been fashionable for decades. Across four subsequent generations, at least four studies have suggested that patients who develop paranoia late in life are likely also to have acquired the sensory deficit of deafness. This is not to say, of course, that people who become deaf are highly likely to develop paranoid thinking—deafness is common, paranoid thinking is not. Besides acquired deafness, the following factors may contribute to the development of late paraphrenia: genetic makeup, a schizotypal personality disorder, menopausal and hormonal changes, and social isolation.

DSM-IV mentions auditory nerve damage in association with paranoia, but there are few supporting studies. And some writers have found an association between congenital deafness and other mental disorders in children. Although the meaning of these associations is as yet unclear, they are there to be found, and we are left to understand them as best we can.

Physical Symptoms

The patient has hearing loss sufficient to interfere with the ability to communicate. This loss may or may not be remediable with a hearing aid.

Mental Symptoms

As compared to younger schizophrenia patients, deaf patients with paranoia have more nonauditory hallucinations, less blunting of affect and more persecutory delusions. They do *not* have formal thought disorder (tangential or otherwise illogical speech). The symptoms are different enough from schizophrenia in younger patients to cause some writers to assert that this late-onset psychosis is a different disorder entirely.

Though less clear-cut, some evidence suggests that children with congenital deafness are more likely to be diagnosed with anxiety disorders such as social phobia and even obsessive compulsive disorder. Deaf children do not appear especially prone to mood or conduct disorders.

Evaluation

Audiometry.

Outlook

According to some reports, patients with late-onset psychosis are more likely than schizophrenia patients to respond completely when treated with antipsychotic medication.

DIABETES MELLITUS

Occurrence	Age of onset	Gender	Refer to
Common	Bimodal	About equal	Endocrinologist
What: Reduced insulin effectiveness or availability causes high blood sugar			
Physical: Increased hunger, thirst, urine output, weight loss, arteriosclerosis			
Mental: Panic attacks, depression, delirium			

Diabetes was probably known to the ancient Egyptians and Greeks, yet we only learned the cause, a deficiency of a substance produced in the pancreas, about 100 years ago. And until 1921, there was no effective treatment for this common, once-deadly disorder, whose effective management seems so routine today.

Insulin is produced in endocrine glands called the islets of Langerhans that are distributed throughout the pancreas. We need insulin to move glucose from the bloodstream into the body's cells. If the insulin is defective or present in inadequate quantities, sugar builds up in the blood and is eventually eliminated through the kidneys. This results in a body that is starved for its usual source of energy and urine that is sweet (diabetes mellitus literally means "honey flowing through").

The more severe form of this illness, insulin-dependent diabetes mellitus (IDDM), is the less common, accounting for perhaps 25% of all diabetes patients. Typically beginning in adolescence or young adulthood, a strong hereditary component renders the pancreas vulnerable to autoimmune destruction of its cells as a response to inflammation. Men and women are about equally affected. Much less commonly, older people may develop IDDM as a complication of chronic alcoholism or other causes.

Non-insulin-dependent diabetes (NIDDM) is a less severe illness of later adulthood. It also runs in families and is likely to occur in people who are obese, but no one knows exactly why these people get the disease. Together, the two types of diabetes affect around 1% of the general population and constitute the most frequently encountered of all the endocrine disorders.

Physical Symptoms

In diabetes that is out of control, the kidneys work hard to eliminate excess sugar from the blood. The patient urinates a great deal and so experiences thirst. Because so much energy-producing glucose is lost, appetite also increases. Besides the three classic early symptoms of thirst, increased eating, and excessive urination, the patient will also lose weight. Damage to peripheral nerves may produce complaints of burning pains (paresthesias) of the legs or feet. Impotence can be a problem; occasionally it is the presenting complaint of a man (or his spouse). It is usually not until years later that diabetic people develop the arteriosclerotic consequences of diabetes—blindness, kidney damage, and blockage of tiny blood vessels in the extremities, which can lead to amputations.

Mental Symptoms

A large number—perhaps two-thirds—of patients with diabetes also have mental disorders. Foremost among these are major depressive and anxiety disorders. Once the diabetic patient has begun treatment, it is unusual for transient high blood sugar levels to cause mental symptoms. But low blood sugar levels (hypoglycemia), such as occur with too much injected insulin, often produce mental symptomatology. As the blood sugar level dips below 40, the patient may notice symptoms that resemble a panic attack: anxiety, dizziness, rapid pulse, and sweating with lightheadedness. There may also be somatic symptoms such as hunger, double or blurred vision, loss of coordination, or difficulty speaking clearly. Although children may have seizures, they are rare in adults.

Even if they escape total impotence, men may experience a loss of sex interest and decreased arousal and enjoyment of sex. Young diabetic women sometimes develop eating disorders (anorexia nervosa and bulimia nervosa), greatly complicating management of diabetes. High blood sugar can cause delirium, which, if prolonged, could conceivably result in dementia.

Evaluation

That old standby, the glucose tolerance test, in which blood sugars are drawn at intervals after a standard "meal" of glucose, may overdiagnose diabetes. Even a patient's anxiety about having blood drawn can produce an abnormal test. The diagnosis of diabetes mellitus should require abnormal blood test results on at least two separate occasions.

Outcome

Within living memory, before the advent of insulin therapy, severe diabetes mellitus meant death within a few years. Now, with careful management, patients enjoy full life spans with modest inconvenience.

Note on Hypoglycemia

Besides occurring as a reaction to insulin or the oral medications used to control diabetes, low blood sugar can be caused by a variety of other conditions. These include severe alcoholism, tumors of the pancreas, and surgery that removes part of the digestive tract. But a major dispute has existed for many years about the diagnosis of reactive hypoglycemia, in which within a few hours of eating a meal patients complain of many of the previously listed symptoms. Although it is likely that in some patients a physiological basis exists for such symptoms, objective studies prove negative for the vast majority. Reactive hypoglycemia has become another of those diagnoses of convenience, used by some clinicians who have no better thoughts on how to classify patients.

EPILEPSY

Occurrence	Age of onset	Gender	Refer to
Common	First three decades	Nearly equal	Neurologist
What: Seizures due to disorder of brain structure			
Physical: Synchronous muscle contractions, with or without loss of consciousness			
Mental: Depression, completed suicide, paranoid psychosis, mental retardation, personality traits, problems of living			

Was there ever a serious disease that has affected a larger number of famous people? In a bibliography entitled *Diseases of Famous People,** just over 10% of the 380 historical individuals surveyed allegedly had had a seizure disorder—second in numbers only to tuberculosis. Known to the ancients (Aristotle) as "the falling sickness," the diagnosis of epilepsy has been ascribed to famous people as disparate as Julius Caesar, Mohammed, and

---

*Submitted by Helen R. Potter, RN, in 1965, as Master's thesis to the Catholic University of America, Washington, D.C.

Joan of Arc. Literature has been shaped by writers with the disease, including Fyodor Dostoyevsky and, probably, Gustave Flaubert, Lord Byron, and Edward Lear. It is even more deserving than hemophilia to be called the "disease of kings," having affected Louis XIII (France), Charles V (Spain), Alexander the Great (Macedonia), Peter the Great (Russia), and William III (England). (It has also been suggested as the disease of Amenhotep IV of Egypt. But because he reigned about 3,400 years ago, the evidence is a bit remote.)

A seizure is a synchronized, rapid discharge of brain neurons that leads to abnormalities of behavior or thinking. This broad definition covers a number of types of seizure disorder, but only two of them have much relevance in the context of this book. They are grand mal and complex partial seizures. Altogether, about 1% of the general population has epilepsy.

Physical Symptoms

Temporal lobe epilepsy, or complex partial seizure, is the most frequently occurring of the seizure disorders. Often caused by a high fever in infancy, at times by brain trauma, hypoxia, or viral infection, these seizures usually (but not always) begin in the temporal lobe of the brain. Though they usually begin suddenly, the patient does not fall to the ground or completely pass out but may experience altered levels of consciousness and bizarre behavior.

Though they are less common, grand mal seizures are probably most familiar to the general public. These typically begin with an aura (usually a smell, sound, or other premonitory sensation) that rapidly gives way to loss of consciousness, falling to the ground, and tonic–clonic motions of skeletal muscles. Involuntary tongue-biting, urination, or defecation may occur. The patient is amnesic for the episode and drowsy for minutes or hours afterward.

Mental Symptoms

Depressive disorders are extremely common, affecting perhaps half of epilepsy patients. However, because of atypical features and "organic" symptoms, most patients probably don't qualify for major depressive disorder. Mania is rare, though not unheard of. The suicide rate is at least five times that of the general population, and according to some authorities, it is even more common in patients with complex partial seizures.

Psychosis, which is found in up to 7% of epilepsy patients, may be brief or long-standing. When the former, hallucinations or delusions may occur during seizures or, in some cases, during the periods of time in between them (called interictal psychosis). All manner of psychotic symptom, including catatonia and the negative symptoms of blunted affect and avolition, have been reported.

Better seizure control usually reduces the severity of the psychotic symptoms. However, paranoid psychosis, with symptoms remarkably similar to paranoid schizophrenia, occurs in some patients, beginning around 14 years after symptoms of complex partial seizures first appear. (You can see why I haven't used abbreviations: CPS stands for complex partial seizures and for chronic paranoid schizophrenia, not to mention cycles per second.) In this case, the paranoid symptoms do not usually abate with adequate treatment of the seizure disorder.

Over the course of a century or more, other mental syndromes have been reported by various authors. Loss of sexual interest is frequent, and not only when epileptic patients become depressed. Mental retardation is also common, usually stemming from the same factor (e.g., cerebral palsy) that initiated the seizures themselves. However, only rarely do epilepsy patients suffer from a deteriorating dementia.

Personality disorder has been reported by many authors. The trouble is, well-controlled studies often do *not* find any particular personality type to be characteristic of epilepsy patients. Those that do, report that borderline personality disorder is common; so is a set of personality traits that includes tenacity, humorlessness, overinclusive thinking, and a marked interest in philosophical or religious matters. Rather than personality disorder, it is probably much more common for patients to have problems of living, the source of which is often social stigma that result from having a brain that intermittently malfunctions.

Finally, be alert for the development of pseudoseizures. Of course, they can occur as conversion symptoms in patients who do not have epilepsy at all. But many patients who have genuine "organic" (to use pre-DSM-IV terminology) seizures also have some seizures that can be shown by EEG to be factitious—faked, either consciously or unconsciously. Why this should occur is probably best understood by considering the personality and life circumstances of the individual patient.

Evaluation

EEG is the most widely used laboratory measure; when recorded during a seizure episode, it will usually be diagnostic. Of course, patients who develop a seizure disorder after the age of 30 must be evaluated with special care for other causes of brain pathology, such as tumors.

Outlook

In some cases, epilepsy remits spontaneously. Even when severe, most patients can be effectively treated with anticonvulsant medications. An occasional patient will require surgery to ablate the trigger area of the brain from which the seizures originate. Epilepsy patients sometimes come to grief when a clinician encounters seizures that are not genuine and assumes that all of their seizures are concocted.

FIBROMYALGIA

Occurrence	Age of onset	Gender	Refer to
See text	25–45	Females predominate	See text

What: Ill-defined cluster of symptoms that may constitute a medical disorder
Physical: Muscle pain, stiffness, tenderness
Mental: Chronic fatigue, depression/dysthymia, anxiety

If you're one of those people who avoids controversy like a dirty needle, better skip this section. There is practically nothing about this topic that is clear-cut, agreed upon by experts, or stable.

This condition, which has only been recognized during the past few years, may occur in up to 5% of the general population, though one study reports that, using strict criteria, only 1 patient could be identified in over 13,000. When it occurs at all, it usually affects young women, though it has also been reported in children. No one knows the cause, though some have suggested that it could be related to the deprivation of non-REM sleep. Despite the fact that another name for it is fibrositis, the muscles do not become inflamed (in fact, there is no discernible pathology at all). Some writers believe that this disorder is due to an abnormality of the patient's immune system.

Various authors have argued that it precedes, or is caused by, or has no particular association with mental disorders. Indeed, this is a condition that appears better accepted by medical clinicians than by mental health professionals, a fact that should give us all pause.

Physical Symptoms

However, authorities do generally agree as to the physical manifestations of fibromyalgia. These include muscle pain, which is generalized; stiffness of the hips, shoulders, and trunk, especially upon awakening; and tenderness that is often exquisite. Such tenderness can affect a number of points upon the body, including the base of the skull, the lower part of the neck, the top of the shoulders, and others, for a total of 18 in all. Although the current research definition requires that a patient identify tenderness in at least 11 of these points, many patients will report fewer, yet receive the clinical diagnosis anyway. Although patients complain of swollen joints, these complaints cannot be validated by objective measurements.

Migraine headaches, irritable bowel syndrome, and dysmenorrhea (painful menses) are prominent among the medical disorders that have been associated with this condition.

Mental Symptoms

Many, but by no means all, patients report emotional problems, which may or may not antedate the onset of physical symptoms. (The science is still a little tender here, folks.) These patients awaken tired, with the complaint that sleep is not refreshing. The most commonly reported symptom is easy fatigability, and there appears to be strong overlap of symptoms and demographics among sufferers of fibromyalgia and the chronic fatigue syndrome.

The commonly associated mental syndromes are mood disorders (especially major depressive disorder, but also dysthymia). In some patients, brief periods of high mood that may not qualify for hypomania can occur. Anxiety symptoms are also reported, including instances of full-blown panic attacks. A few studies have reported cognitive disabilities that do not reach the degree needed for a diagnosis of dementia or delirium: slowed performance of psychomotor tasks, inattention, memory deficits. Patients may lack initiative and have dependent or obsessive–compulsive personality traits.

In at least one study, many patients were found to have somatization disorder. This finding would be consistent with the age of onset, sex distribution, and, especially, the elusive nature of this puzzling condition.

Evaluation

Unhappily (and, to my mind, somewhat suspiciously), no laboratory studies have been identified that can help pinpoint the diagnosis.

Outlook

There seems to be little consensus about prognosis. One study found about two-thirds of patients improved on follow-up, though few cures. But some patients continue symptomatic and disabled for many years. Some clinicians would argue that the outcome will depend on how well the underlying mental condition can be addressed.

HEAD TRAUMA

Occurrence	Age of onset	Gender	Refer to
Common	Especially 15–24	Males predominate	Neurologist
What: Nonpenetrating injury to the brain produces temporary or permanent symptoms			
Physical: Headache, dizziness, fatigue, paralysis, anosmia, seizures			
Mental: Amnesia, personality change, delirium, dementia, mood swings, anxiety, psychosis			

In any given year in the United States, around 2 million people experience head trauma. (It should come as no surprise that men outnumber women by about two to one.) Most of those cases are not too serious, or we'd be awash in donor kidneys and corneas. Although nearly one-fourth of these patients initially require hospitalization, only about 4% develop permanent disability. However, many of the rest do have some sort of resulting mental problems, often with attendant physical symptoms.

In this section, I'll discuss several types of head injury and the problems that can result. I will limit the discussion, however, to closed head injuries—those that do not penetrate the brain. Obviously, open head injuries have the potential for consequences that are even more devastating. And of course, what makes brain trauma at once fascinating and frightening is that, unlike so many of the conditions reported in this book, it could happen to any one of us at any time.

Based on the nature and degree of damage to the brain's tissues, there are any number of ways to describe brain injuries. But some syndromes are so common that nearly everyone knows someone who has been affected by one. Because there are several groups of symptoms to describe here, I'm going to step outside my usual format.

Concussion

This common term denotes a sudden, brief loss of consciousness immediately following a blow to the head. The patient feels dazed, for a moment or two is unresponsive, and almost always suffers some degree of amnesia, usually for the period just before the injury occurred (called retrograde amnesia). This loss of memory may last for a few minutes to several days, or even weeks. In mild cases, the amnesia lasts less than a day; the more severe the injury, the longer the interval of amnesia. It is rare, though not unheard of, for memory subsequent to the injury to be affected; this type is termed anterograde amnesia. There are usually no pathological changes in the brain tissues, and there are no laboratory exams that might help with the diagnosis. The outlook for complete recovery is excellent, though headache may persist for a while.

Postconcussion Syndrome

Although most concussion patients recover rapidly, many experience a variable period of fatigue, dizziness, some memory impairment, and poor concentration. There is usually headache that resembles tension headache—at the front and base of the skull. Patients sometimes complain of problems with sleep or loss of interest in sex. These symptoms usually begin shortly after the injury and last for 8 or 10 weeks; however, there are many reports of patients who have continued to have symptoms for years.

The patient (or family) may note personality changes of apathy and loss of spontaneity. Depression, anxiety, and irritability are other hallmarks. Recent studies suggest that patients are more likely to develop postconcussion syndrome if they have had social problems, such as divorce and job dislocations, prior to the injury.

Contusion

The term contusion simply means that there has been bruising of any part of the body that has soft tissue. The bruise usually appears at one of two places: just under the point of impact, or at a point on the side of the skull opposite the blow. The second type, called contrecoup, occurs when the brain, accelerated in the direction of the blow, in effect bounces off the other side of the skull. In either case, there is loss of consciousness.

Contusions are more serious than concussions; at the site of bruising occur tiny areas of bleeding, with some tissue destruction. The physical symptoms can be more serious, too, ranging from persistent, severe headache to paralysis or even coma. Not uncommonly there is disruption of the olfactory tracts, which are located in an exposed location on the underside of the frontal lobes. When this happens, patients lose their ability to detect odors. Because so much of taste rests with the sense of smell, such patients also complain that food no longer tastes good.

Besides amnesia, personality change is especially likely in contusion—the same sort of syndrome that you might find in any other severe head injury. It is said that brain injuries accentuate any previous personality characteristics, but two principal syndromes have been identified: taciturnity and aggression.

Injury to the frontal lobes is especially likely to result in a quiet, or taciturn demeanor, with loss of motivation and lowered energy level; abulia (the loss of willpower, or the ability to make decisions) is also encountered. Some patients may not even recognize that they are impaired (anosognosia). Other patients with frontal lobe injury may instead lose previous inhibitions, becoming impulsive and excitable; they may have difficulty focusing attention on a task; relatives and friends may be embarrassed by their socially inappropriate behavior.

Temporal lobe injuries can spark the tendency to pathological aggression; such emotionally unstable patients may easily fly off the handle, sometimes even exploding in rage. Other characteristics sometimes described in temporal lobe patients include preoccupation with somatic symptoms, perhaps to the point of hypochondriasis.

Other than personality change, a variety of mental disorders can result from contusion. Depression is perhaps one of the most common. Although the symptoms are identical to those of endogenous depression (e.g., major depressive disorder or bipolar I disorder, most recent episode depressive), relatively brief (up to 2 months) secondary manias have also been reported in nearly 10% of patients. Psychosis has also been found, even after relatively mild brain injury.

Other Brain Injury Syndromes

Delirium frequently develops, regardless of the severity of injury. Although the difficulty in maintaining attention and processing information is often relatively short-lived, some patients develop more severe symptoms and eventually are diagnosed as suffering from dementia. Of course, the greater the original brain injury, the more extensive we might expect the mental consequences to be. But deep, confluent contusions will present with such disabling symptoms (paralysis, coma) that mental health professionals are at little risk for having to make the initial diagnosis in such a patient.

Several other terms come up in describing the effects of closed brain trauma.

Subdural Hematoma

Resulting from a head injury that may be severe, but perhaps resulting from only a glancing blow, this is the accumulation of a pool of blood between the surface of the brain and its tough, membranous covering, the dura mater. Though small subdural hematomas may produce no symptoms at all, larger ones produce symptoms by taking up space normally occupied by brain tissue. The acute effects are usually drowsiness, with a one-sided headache; the pupil of the eye on that same side may be enlarged. Coma often supervenes.

Weeks or months after the injury, some patients develop symptoms of chronic subdural hematoma. (About one-fourth of these patients report no history of head injury at all.) Characteristic is headache that fluctuates in severity or with changes in position. Seizures and a paresis (partial paralysis) on one side of the body can also occur. Mentally, these patients may suffer from disorientation, inattention, drowsiness, or slowed thinking that suggest a delirium; some of the changes in personality encountered in contusion may also occur.

Epidural Hematoma

This is a collection of blood between the dura and skull. Mental changes occur much more rapidly than in subdurals, and there may be a period of lucidity before coma sets in.

Evaluation

Skull X-rays will usually reveal a fracture in epidural hematomas. CT scans or MRI may be necessary to visualize contusions, or subdural hematomas but will reveal no evidence of brain pathology at all in concussion.

Outlook

As you might imagine, prognosis will be extremely variable. Most concussion patients suffer no permanent effects, though some will be bothered for a variable time if they have postconcussion syndrome. For some, postconcussion syndrome has been reported to be chronically disabling. In addition to cognitive problems, those with personality change may experience problems with substance abuse, inappropriate aggression, and the too-free expression of sexual urges. The outcome of contusions depends on the location and extent of injury, as well as on the age of the patient. Due to the plasticity of their brains, children are most likely to recover completely, though very young children and the elderly reportedly fare worse than others.

HERPES ENCEPHALITIS

Occurrence	Age of onset	Gender	Refer to
Uncommon	Childhood and middle age	Females predominate slightly	Infectious disease specialist
What: Infection of brain by herpes virus			
Physical: Fever, headache, stiff neck, vomiting, focal neurological symptoms			
Mental: Forgetfulness, anxiety, psychosis			

The number of ways a person can experience a brain infection may not be exactly endless, but there are certainly many opportunities. They can all be reduced to just a few main categories, however; at least one section of this book is devoted to an example of each (at the page numbers indicated):

- Slow viruses (HIV disease, p. 47)
- Acute viral encephalitis (herpes, pp. 96–98)
- Chronic bacterial infections (syphilis, p. 174, and Lyme disease, p. 123)
- Prions (Creutzfeldt–Jakob disease, p. 160)
- Fungi (cryptococcosis, p. 78)
- Parasites (pretty rare in the United States; not discussed here)

Of the causes of acute viral encephalitis, herpes is perhaps the most common, affecting perhaps 2 or 3 people per 1 million each year. Milder degrees of behavioral and mental disturbances can be found with other causes of encephalitis, such as mumps. The distribution of cases across the general population is bimodal: ages 5–30 and over 50 are the two groups most affected.

Physical Symptoms

Onset is usually rapid, heralded by abrupt onset of fever and headache, and sometimes by seizures. Responding poorly to aspirin, temperature hovers in the range of 101–104 degrees. Signs of meningitis (stiff neck, vomiting) frequently occur. Focal neurological signs may include paralysis of half the body (hemiparesis), the inability to recognize objects (aphasia), and numbness or tingling (paresthesias) of the buttocks or perineal areas. Other symptoms include constipation, impotence, and urinary retention.

Mental Symptoms

Early in the course of the disease may be noted cognitive changes, including loss of memory, difficulty organizing things, and trouble naming things. For example, a patient may selectively be unable to recall the names of specific plants. Some patients have developed psychosis; others have developed the Klüver–Bucy syndrome, a rare condition that combines placid temperament, excessive eating and interest in sex, and use of the mouth to examine objects. Patients with encephalitis have also reported anxiety symptoms; rarely, one encounters symptoms of catatonia.

Evaluation

Most patients will have an abnormal EEG (diffuse or focal slow brain waves, sharp waves over the sides of the brain). Once the disorder has progressed for a week or more, CT scan may also show abnormalities. However, the definitive diagnosis needed to institute therapy may be possible only with a brain biopsy.

Outlook

Though the disorder is treatable with modern, virus-fighting drugs, herpes encephalitis still kills about two-thirds of its victims. Most survivors will have serious residual symptoms. Especially common are dementia, aphasia, and amnesia. Some will only be bothered by weakness of the legs for months after recovery.

HOMOCYSTINURIA

Occurrence	Age of onset	Gender	Refer to
Uncommon	Childhood	Equal	Endocrinologist
What: Inborn error of metabolism allows accumulation of homocysteine and methionine			
Physical: Impaired vision, shuffling gait, blotchy skin			
Mental: Mental retardation, dementia, behavioral problems			

The human race is afflicted with seemingly countless inborn errors of metabolism, which are inherited defects in the way one chemical substance is converted to another. Homocystinuria is an error in the metabolism of protein that allows two amino acids, homocysteine and methionine, to accumulate in the body's fluids and tissues. (It can actually result from any of seven separate metabolic errors, all of which can cause symptoms—and more pathways could be discovered in the future.) Despite their number, the overall effect is still small. Worldwide, only about 1 in 200,000 individuals has homocystinuria. Why it should be five times more common in Ireland is only one of the Emerald Isle's enduring mysteries.

Physical Symptoms

The disorder usually manifests itself early; exact symptoms depend on which of the seven forms of this disorder the individual has inherited. As small children, over three-fourths of these patients develop glaucoma and impaired vision from dislocation of the lens of the eye. There are red blotches on the skin over the cheeks, and hair tends to be brittle and sparse. Gait is marked by shuffling. Blood clots form in arteries that nourish the brain, heart, and kidneys; the symptoms that result are what you might expect from the death of all or parts of these organs (paralyses, focal symptoms).

Mental Symptoms

Half or more of these patients will have mental retardation, which is usually relatively mild. Some will have ill-defined behavioral abnormalities; still others become demented relatively early in life. A catatonic syndrome has been reported in one form of homocystinuria; this is exceedingly rare, however.

Evaluation

Special chemical tests of the blood or urine will reveal elevated levels of the amino acids mentioned earlier. Such tests are not exactly routine, however; clinicians only order them if they already suspect the diagnosis.

Outlook

Like so much else in healthcare, how well the patient does depends on how soon therapy is started. With early diagnosis, the clinician will know which amino acids require dietary restriction or supplementation. There have even been reports of patients whose catatonia has been successfully treated with folate, which catalyzes one of the chemical steps in the production of amino acids. Still, death from vascular disease by age 30 is the fate of nearly one-fourth of these patients.

HUNTINGTON'S DISEASE

Occurrence	Age of onset	Gender	Refer to
Uncommon	By late 30s	Equal	Neurologist
What: Inherited, fatal neurological disease that has no cure			
Physical: Writing motions of limbs, ataxia, inarticulate speech			
Mental: Depression, psychosis, personality change (apathy, disinhibition), dementia			

One of the icons of my generation, and that of my parents, was the fabled guitar player, singer, and composer Woody Guthrie. Named for Woodrow Wilson, he lived with hoboes in the 1930s and wrote over 1,000 songs, including such folk classics as "Union Maid," and "So Long, It's Been Good to Know Yuh." Probably his most famous, "This Land Is Your Land," was taken up as a sort of unofficial theme song by the Civil Rights movement in the 1960s. The last few years of his life, he did not play at all, however, but rather was confined to a hospital bed in New York, the victim of Huntington's disease. He died there in 1967, at age 55.

Years ago, it was called Huntington's chorea, but it is now generally recognized that the symptoms entail problems far beyond the involuntary, purposeless, writhing movements that constitute the neurological syndrome of chorea. Huntington's disease is inherited as an autosomal dominant with 100% penetrance. This genetic jargon means that the son or daughter of an affected mother or father has a 50% chance of inheriting the gene, and anyone who does so—and lives long enough—is sure to develop symptoms. The gene causes atrophy of the caudate nucleus, a large group of cells shaped roughly like a question mark, buried deep within the substance of the brain.

The prevalence is around 8 per 100,000 population. Although all races and cultures can be affected, Caucasians are at greatest risk; among Japanese, the disease occurs only about one-tenth as often. Although onset usually occurs in early adult life (by the late 30s), it has occasionally been reported in childhood. Then, progression is even more rapid than usual, with death occurring in 6–8 years.

In recent years scientists have learned that the genetic underpinning of Huntington's disease is a sequence of DNA nucleotides on chromosome 4 that has been repeated many more times than would be necessary for the normal gene. The phenomenon of genetic anticipation (more severe disease, or earlier age of onset in the children than in parents with the disease) may be due to a greater degree of DNA nucleotide replication in successive generations.

Physical Symptoms

The first indications of this horrible disease may be only an unwonted clumsiness. The patient may fidget more than usual or experience other involuntary physical movements, which can be as slight as a shrugging of the shoulders. At first the patient may try to convert these little movements to purposeful ones, so as to hide their involuntary nature. As the disease inexorably progresses, abrupt and purposeless motions of face, limbs, and trunk develop. Speech becomes inarticulate; swallowing is an effort. Hands and arms twist and point uncontrollably, and at random; the gait, for as long as the patient can still walk, assumes a peculiar gliding quality that sometimes seems almost like dancing. These physical symptoms are worsened by emotion and disappear during sleep.

Mental Symptoms

Early on, there is often depression, which may even precede the first physical symptoms. Around half of Huntington's disease patients have depression to some degree, and many will have a major depressive episode, sometimes with melancholia or delusions. (Then, the appropriate diagnosis, of course, would be depression due to Huntington's disease.) A few patients may be initially psychotic, with delusions or hallucinations, usually auditory. A very small percentage will have manic episodes that can exactly mimic those of bipolar mood disorder.

Another early mental symptom may be that of personality change, which usually takes one of two forms. Some patients will become apathetic and withdraw from ordinary social activities, or neglect grooming or other aspects of hygiene. Others become disinhibited; with unprovoked angry or irritable moods that come and go unpredictably, they may lash out verbally or physically. Some clinicians consider personality change to be one of the defining features of Huntington's disease.

But the most typical mental symptom of all is dementia. Nearly all Huntington's disease patients eventually become demented, and for some, cognitive decline begins early in the course of illness. The patient may first notice an inability to recall information learned earlier or difficulty thinking through the solution to a problem. Cognitive ability declines further as the movement disorder worsens. Psychosis may supervene; by late in the course of illness, around one-third of all patients will have had some psychotic features.

Evaluation

For the patient with typical symptoms and a positive family history, further evaluation is hardly necessary. Genetic testing is available for the occasional patient with early symptoms or for whom an adequate family history is not available (e.g., a parent died at an early age before symptoms developed.)

Outlook

Only the rare patient is spared the ultimate decline into bedridden dementia, mute and unable even to recognize friends or family. About 6% of patients take their own lives, but death usually results from intercurrent infection or choking on food. Their children, half of whom will inherit the responsible gene, can be tested to determine whether they, too, are affected. What they learn can be the ultimate in reprieves, for good news means that neither they nor their offspring will ever have to worry about Huntington's again. But for the other half, the news will be devastating. It is small wonder that many choose not to take the test at all.

HYPERPARATHYROIDISM

Occurrence	Age of onset	Gender	Refer to
Frequent (especially in elderly)	Young adult to old age	Females predominate	Endocrinologist
What: Overactive parathyroid glands cause increase in serum calcium			
Physical: Weakness, tiredness, anorexia, nausea, vomiting, constipation, thirst, abdominal and muscle pain			
Mental: Personality change, depression, suicidal ideas, anxiety, delirium, psychosis			

The parathyroids are four glands, each a bit smaller than a pencil eraser, that nestle behind the thyroid gland, two on either side of the neck. Their job is to regulate the amount of calcium in your system. When the parathyroids work too hard, which happens in perhaps 1 out of 1,000 adults, serum calcium rises. This condition is called hyperparathyroidism, and it sometimes produces symptoms. Nowadays, the condition is often asymptomatic. This is because of the routine use in the United States and other Western countries of blood chemistry screening tests. Disorders such as this one are diagnosed before they can produce symptoms.

In around four out of five patients, the condition is caused by a benign tumor (adenoma) of a parathyroid gland. Incidence peaks around ages 20–40. Taking into account undetected cases, perhaps 1% of all elderly individuals may be affected. Women outnumber men about two to one.

Physical Symptoms

The effect of hyperparathyroidism is to leach calcium out of places that it should be (e.g., bones) and deposit it as stones in places where it shouldn't be (e.g., the kidneys or bladder). Early symptoms include muscle weakness and wasting, tiredness, loss of appetite, nausea and vomiting, constipation, thirst, abdominal pain, and muscle pain. Later, there may be sensory losses, including the inability to smell (anosmia) or stocking-glove anesthesia.

Mental Symptoms

The onset of hyperparathyroidism is usually gradual; mental symptoms may eventually affect half or more of patients, especially those who are elderly. Milder symptoms include personality change, for example, a loss of initiative or decreased spontaneity. Later mental symptoms may resemble mood disorder: apathy, mental depression, anxiety, irritability, and even suicidal ideas at times.

As the patient worsens, symptoms suggestive of cognitive disorder may ensue, including the subjective sensation of slowed mentation, emotional lability, poor concentration, and loss of recent memory. This may eventually result in a classic picture of an agitated delirium. Some patients become psychotic, with persecutory ideas, auditory and visual hallucinations, and even catatonic symptoms. As the serum calcium level climbs even higher, stupor and coma may result. As you might deduce from these symptoms, hyperparathyroidism can be misdiagnosed as somatoform disorder, mood disorder, schizophrenia, or cognitive disorder.

Special Note on Causation

Patients who have been on long-term lithium treatment can have symptoms that closely resemble those of hyperparathyroidism.

Evaluation

Measure serum calcium, parathyroid hormone.

Outcome

Surgical removal of the hyperactive parathyroid gland will cure 90–95% of patients. After treatment, even demented elderly patients may improve in their ability to perform activities of daily living. Even without intervention, milder degrees of hyperparathyroidism can be quite benign and last for years or a lifetime without producing symptoms. (In such an instance, one might ask, Is this really a disease?)

HYPERTENSIVE ENCEPHALOPATHY

Occurrence	Age of onset	Gender	Refer to
Frequent	40s	Males predominate	Internist, urgently
What: High blood pressure causes pathological brain changes			
Physical: Headache, nausea, vomiting, seizures, paralysis, visual impairment			
Mental: Delirium, paranoia			

Thirty percent of adult Americans have high blood pressure. This should come as no surprise, considering that over one-third of us are overweight. No one quite understands why obesity encourages hypertension, but the effects are quite clear: stroke and cardiovascular disease. Of course, most patients who have hypertension do not have obvious mental symptoms (though studies have shown that even when high blood pressure is well controlled, patients don't do as well as nonhypertensive people on tests of attention and memory).

But about 1 in 100 hypertensive patients has an extremely severe form of the disease, known as malignant hypertension. It sounds bad, and it is. Blood pressure rises to a level high enough (above 130 mm diastolic) and long enough that swelling and multiple small thrombi (blood clots) develop in the brain substance itself, thus causing the symptoms of hypertensive encephalopathy. This disorder occurs more commonly in men and begins at the relatively early average age of about 40. Black people are more likely than Whites to have malignant hypertension. Untreated, it leads rapidly to death and should be considered a true medical emergency.

Physical Symptoms

Mostly, hypertension is silent: The vast majority of patients have no symptoms at all. It is only when hypertension becomes severe that symptoms develop, even including headache. Headache is the symptom most typical of hypertension; when it does occur, it is usually at the back of the head (occipital). Hemorrhages on the surface of the retina lead to blurring of vision and other visual disturbances, even blindness. Other symptoms include dizziness, heart palpitations, nausea and vomiting, seizures, paralysis, tiredness, and sometimes impotence.

Mental Symptoms

These wax and wane. Most often, they take a form of delirium characterized by a decrease in alertness that may be experienced as only drowsiness, but can progress to stupor or coma. Patients may feel slowed mentally, become easily confused (disoriented), and experience loss of recent memory. Paranoid psychosis has occasionally been reported.

Evaluation

Little outside the simple measurement of blood pressure by using a sphygmomanometer (the gadget they pump up on your arm) is necessary to establish the fact of severe hypertension. But a variety of additional tests may be required to rule out treatable causes such as pheochromocytoma and kidney disease.

Outlook

Often suffering kidney and heart disease as well, these are among the most severely ill of medical patients. Yet, once blood pressure has been brought under control, physical and mental symptoms will usually abate.

HYPERTHYROIDISM

Occurrence	Age of onset	Gender	Refer to
Common	20–40	Females predominate	Endocrinologist
What: Overactive thyroid gland produces excessive thyroid hormone			
Physical: Goiter, bulging eyes, weakness, palpitations, hunger, weight loss, tremor, diarrhea, warm skin			
Mental: Agitated or apathetic depression, anxiety, panic attacks, delirium, psychosis			

Of all the disorders included in this book, hyperthyroidism is one of the most important for mental health clinicians. Why? Because it is common (affecting as many as 3 patients per 10,000 women per year), serious, easily mistaken for a variety of primary mental disorders, yet, in most cases, easily treatable. If you only achieve familiarity with a few medical disorders, let one of them be this one!

In hyperthyroidism, the thyroid gland produces too much of one of its hormones, thyroxine. This hormone regulates metabolic activity in all of the body's tissues, including the central nervous system. Too much thyroxine increases metabolic rate, creating symptoms (thyrotoxicosis) that affect nearly every organ system.

Graves' disease, with attendant thyrotoxicosis symptoms, is the most common form of hyperthyroidism, accounting for perhaps 80% of cases. Another important cause of hyperthyroidism is taking too much prescription thyroxine, either in a too-vigorous attempt to correct a hypothyroid condition or, sometimes, in an effort to lose weight.

Hyperthyroidism can occur at any age, but it most often begins between the ages of 20 and 40. By a ratio of 3 or 4 to 1, it is a woman's disease. Graves' disease may be familial.

Physical Symptoms

One of the most characteristic and obvious outward signs of hyperthyroidism is the goiter, the characteristic enlargement of the thyroid gland that appears as a swelling on the sides of the lower neck. Hyperthyroid patients also complain of rapid heart-beat and palpitations of the heart. They may lose weight despite an increase in appetite. They sweat excessively, have warm skin, and complain bitterly that they *feel* too warm, leading to thermostat wars with relatives. Their hair becomes fine-textured. They may also experience shortness of breath, frequent bowel movements, and reduced menstrual flow.

More severely ill patients may show a variety of eye signs: exophthalmos (bulging of the eye ball from the socket), staring gaze, decreased rate of blinking, lid lag (there is a delay in the descent of the upper eyelid as the patient directs the gaze downward). There may be wasting of the large, flat muscle of the temple, producing a sunken appearance to the sides of the head, or of the thighs, causing severely ill patients to have difficulty climbing stairs and to complain of weakness. In severe cases, the skin over the shins may become darker and thicker, somewhat resembling the peel of an orange. There may also be a fine tremor of the hands.

Mental Symptoms

Younger patients, especially, may complain of depression or nervousness, and may show an increased lability of mood. Restless, irritable, and complaining of nervousness, they may have trouble sleeping and feel fatigued much of the time. They will sometimes be treated for an agitated depression. Anxiety symptoms may suggest panic disorder, generalized anxiety disorder, or social phobia. When very severe, delirium with profound agitation and psychotic symptoms can ensue.

In elderly patients, the picture may more resemble an apathetic depression; these patients complain principally of tiredness and heartbeat irregularities.

Evaluation

A serum thyroxine (T4) level will be elevated, and the thyroid stimulating hormone (TSH) will be decreased. More exotic tests may be needed to determine the exact cause of the hyperthyroidism.

Outcome

With appropriate treatment (usually medication or radioactive iodine, but occasionally surgery), most patients will completely recover from their symptoms. Unrecognized, hence untreated, hyperthyroidism can lead to cardiac enlargement and eventual heart failure.

HYPOPARATHYROIDISM

Occurrence	Age of onset	Gender	Refer to
Uncommon (see text)	Young adulthood	Females predominate	Endocrinologist
What: Inadequate parathyroid hormone production causes low serum calcium			
Physical: Numbness and tingling, seizures, spasms of face, hands, feet			
Mental: Irritability, depression, anxiety, paranoid ideas, delirium, dementia			

The single greatest cause of hypoparathyroidism is hyperparathyroidism. This isn't really a paradox, just a consequence of the surgeon's dilemma: When operating on a parathyroid tumor, is it better to remove less tissue and risk continuing hyperparathyroidism, or to remove more tissue and risk leaving the patient with too little remaining gland to function properly? Of course, something in between would be preferable, but even the best surgeons can't hit it right every time. Other, rarer causes of hypoparathyroidism include chronic alcoholism, and autoimmune disorders, and a resistance to parathyroid hormone termed pseudohypoparathyroidism.

For some reason, prevalence data are really hard to come by for this disorder. A bit of extrapolation is in order. Whereas most cases are surgical, less than 2% of neck operations result in hypoparathyroidism. I would therefore categorize the prevalence of this condition as "uncommon." Most patients with either hyperthyroidism or hyperparathyroidism are young adult females, so that is the group that should also be most likely to develop hypoparathyroidism.

Physical Symptoms

The low serum calcium (hypocalcemia) that results from too little parathyroid hormone causes the junctions between nerves and muscles to become overly excitable. Early symptoms can include tingling or numbness of the lips, hands, or feet. More severely ill patients may have facial grimacing or spasms of wrists or ankles. Ultimately, seizures may ensue.

Mental Symptoms

In all, perhaps half of hypoparathyroid patients will have mental symptoms. The severity and extent of the symptoms may be in direct proportion to the rapidity with which serum calcium falls.

As with so many endocrine disorders, there can be a considerable variety of emotional symptoms. Some patients are quite irritable; others are depressed (reportedly, they only rarely express the feelings of guilt that would be typical of a severe major depressive episode); many may show rapidly changing emotions (emotional lability) and anxiety symptoms, including phobias and obsessions. Some evidence suggests that rapidly dropping serum calcium may also provoke more severe symptoms such as paranoid ideas or auditory or visual hallucinations. Patients may become agitated and disoriented, sometimes yielding a picture of delirium.

Severe cognitive difficulties can develop when serum calcium levels remain low for months or longer. Thinking slows and memory declines, eventually producing the social withdrawal of frank dementia. Such serious developments are not often seen in cases of surgical hypoparathyroidism—surgeons and internists are alert to such changes in the days and weeks postoperative.

Evaluation

The screening test is easy: Serum calcium level will be low, as will serum parathyroid hormone.

Tangential Note on Diagnosis

As you will surmise, there is considerable opportunity for misdiagnosis in hypothyroid patients. Their mental symptoms can be confused with mood, anxiety, and psychotic disorders. And twitching of various muscles causes facial grimacing or twisting of the wrist or ankle (called carpopedal spasm) that can be mistaken for conversion symptoms.

Conversion disorder is the DSM-IV somatoform diagnosis that should be reserved as a "last resort" diagnosis to be used only after all physical diagnoses (and other somatoform diagnoses) have been considered and rejected. In my view, when you encounter complaints that look like "conversion symptoms," you should look carefully for other symptoms of somatization disorder. If you cannot substantiate somatization disorder, it is better to call the patient "undiagnosed" than to use the term *conversion disorder*, which has never been proven to have good reliability or validity.

Outlook

Physical and mental symptoms will disappear as treatment with vitamin D and calcium brings serum calcium levels back to normal. However, some degree of intellectual deficit may persist for patients with long-standing dementia. Psychotic symptoms encountered in postparathyroidectomy patients usually remit spontaneously and quickly.

HYPOTHYROIDISM

Occurrence	Age of onset	Gender	Refer to
Common	50–60	Females predominate	Endocrinologist
What: Thyroid produces too little hormone, so body processes generally slow down			
Physical: Slow heartbeat, dry skin, hair loss, edema, weight gain, cold intolerance, goiter			
Mental: Depression, suicidal ideas, mental slowing, apathetic personality change, dementia			

Hypothyroidism is a relatively common disease affecting up to 1% of the general population. It is much more common in older patients, where it may affect 2–4% of the population. But it can occur even in a baby whose mother lacked sufficient iodine in her diet during pregnancy. When it does, and when it is untreated, cretinism is the result.

Cretinism is endemic in mountainous areas of developing countries and even in parts of Europe, where the water does not naturally contain enough iodine. Recently, such has been the case in China, where as many as 10 million children have grown up with varying degrees of mental retardation. Such children typically also have short stature and late puberty. Milder cases may not even be detected until teachers note poor school performance.

In most Western countries, hypothyroidism typically begins late in life. It affects women about three times as often as it does men. In any patient, the onset of symptoms may be so slow as to go undetected by the patient, relatives and, of course, clinicians. But the disease is both common and serious enough that it should be kept in the front of every mental health clinician's mind.

Among mental patients, lithium treatment commonly causes hypothyroidism.

Physical Symptoms

Low levels of thyroxine, the major hormone produced by the thyroid gland, can have profound effects upon many organ systems of the body. Skin may become dry and the hair brittle; sometimes there is a loss of hair from the outer one-third of each eyebrow. Face, feet, and hands may become edematous (puffy), thus accounting for the term myxedema, a synonym for hypothyroidism. As the thyroid gland works harder in its attempt to produce thyroxine, it may become enlarged (goiter). If menses become heavy, as sometimes happens, anemia may develop. The voice may deepen or become hoarse.

Everything seems slowed down in the hypothyroid patient. Appetite falls, but so does metabolism, so weight increases. Heart rate drops, and patients complain of constipation. They also complain bitterly of feeling cold and may be seen wearing sweaters even in the mildest weather. Reflexes (obtained by tapping the tendon just below the kneecap) are also slowed.

Mental Symptoms

Even more often than in its opposite, hy*per*thyroidism, hypothyroid patients complain of feeling depressed, and they may show typical signs and symptoms of major depression. They are apathetic, complain of feeling tired and loss of sex interest. Some will have suicidal ideas. They may complain of poor memory and can even have symptoms such as shortened attention span and slowed thinking that suggest cognitive impairment. Gradual increase in irritability, withdrawal from friends or family, and even suspiciousness may indicate personality change.

Hallucinations or delusions may ensue—"myxedema madness," as it used to be called. However, out-and-out psychosis is an infrequent complication of the disorder. When hypothyroidism is profound or prolonged, patients may even experience stupor. Hypothyroidism is one of the most frequent causes of *reversible* dementia—when it occurs, it usually responds to treatment.

Special Note on Detection

People at particular risk for hypothyroidism are those who have previously had a thyroid ablation procedure (either surgery or chemicals to remove the thyroid gland, or otherwise reduce its output of thyroxine) because of tumors or even hyperthyroidism! As a clue, look for "necklace scars" around the front of the patient's neck. Hypothyroidism is especially prevalent in areas that have a low iodine content in the water—Akron, Ohio, is one of those. Fortunately, nowhere in this country has been so troubled by the ravages of this illness, so serious, yet so treatable, as has modern-day China.

Evaluation

Just the opposite of hy*per*thyroidism, serum thyroxine (T4) level will be decreased and thyroid stimulating hormone (TSH) will be increased. Additional testing may be needed to determine the exact cause of the hypothyroidism.

Outlook

Thyroid replacement therapy is simple, cheap, and often miraculously effective. But even with adequate treatment, patients who suffer long-standing hypothyroidism may not fully recover all areas of cognitive deficit.

KIDNEY FAILURE

Occurrence	Age of onset	Gender	Refer to
Frequent	Varies with cause	Varies with cause	Nephrologist
What: Loss of ability of kidneys to filter waste products from blood			
Physical: Whew! Too numerous for summation; see text			
Mental: Depression			

When acute (e.g., caused by a kidney stone), kidney failure produces few symptoms and is potentially reversible. But chronic kidney (or renal, as it is known in medical circles) failure is a devastatingly serious condition that, even with adequate treatment, can wreak havoc in nearly every organ system of the body. Heart, lung, skin, skeleton, brain, and endocrine glands are all placed at risk for devastation by this pervasive disorder. The collection of symptoms caused by severe renal failure is known as uremia.

Decades ago, a type of kidney infection called glomerulonephritis was the principal villain responsible for kidney failure. Glomerulonephritis has long since yielded to better detection and treatment with antibiotics, so that diabetes and hypertension are now the leading causes of this condition that affects about 1 person in 5,000. Blacks are more likely to be affected than Whites.

All manner of other causes, from congenital disorders such as polycystic kidneys to cancer to the toxic affect of drugs, can produce kidney failure. Author Jack London, in a vain attempt to treat an infectious disease known as yaws, is said to have destroyed his kidneys with the combined effects of copper sulfate, iodoform, boric acid, hydrogen peroxide, Lysol, and a little lime juice, for flavor.

Physical Symptoms

The effect of uremia is a buildup in the blood stream of metabolic waste products that would ordinarily be excreted in the urine. Patients usually don't notice symptoms until the functional capacity of the kidneys drops below 25%. Renal dialysis ameliorates most symptoms but introduces certain problems of its own (see below).

Most patients report decrease in urine output. A partial list of uremia's effects includes the following:

- *Blood.* Anemia (with resulting fatigue), bleeding that is difficult to stop.
- *Skin.* Pallor, bruising, and itching.
- *Gastrointestinal tract.* Upset stomach, loss of appetite, nausea and vomiting, intestinal bleeding (producing black, tarry stools); in severely ill patients, the smell of urine on the breath (termed uremic fetor).
- *Heart.* Congestive heart failure (ankle edema), high blood pressure, and pulmonary edema (with shortness of breath).
- *Skeleton.* With dialysis, spontaneous fractures and bone pain.
- *Metabolic and endocrine systems.* Hypothermia, decreased growth, absent menses, loss of sexual functioning (impotence in most men, decreased female orgasm).
- *Neuromuscular systems.* Lethargy, headaches, muscle irritability (cramps and hiccups), restless legs, unstable gait; when severe, seizures. Neuromuscular symptoms typically fluctuate from one hour or day to the next. Peripheral neuropathy is not distinguishable from neuropathy that is due to diabetes or alcoholism. It is more commonly found in men than in women. Early on, legs are more affected than arms; sensory modalities are more affected than motor. Peripheral neuropathy can progress to paralysis. Restless legs syndrome, a nearly indefinable discomfort of the legs that can be relieved only by moving them, is also quite common, occurring in almost half of patients with

uremia. Asterixis is a characteristic flapping tremor that is best observed by asking the patient to hold both hands outstretched in front as if signaling "stop." The flapping motion at fingers or wrists will begin presently, after an interval of up to 30 seconds.

Mental Symptoms

The mental symptoms derive from uremic encephalopathy (meaning, literally, "brain disease"). As the load of toxins increases, the patient becomes drowsy and inattentive. Delirium ensues; there may be illusions or hallucinations. Memory and judgment begin to slide, and a stupor may develop.

Many of the mental symptoms of chronic renal failure are similar to those of a major depressive episode: poor appetite, insomnia, lethargy. Even in milder cases, patients may feel depressed. Suicide is certainly more common in renal patients than in the general population.

Two other syndromes are related to renal dialysis. Dialysis disequilibrium occurs especially during a patient's first several dialyses and is related to the rapid reduction of the level of urea in the blood. The syndrome comprises nausea, vomiting, headache, drowsiness, and sometimes even seizures. Some patients experience delirium. The symptoms usually last only a few hours or less.

Much more serious is dialysis dementia, which develops after several years of frequent dialysis. Patients experience trouble speaking, twitching motions of muscle groups (called myoclonus), seizures, dementia, and, eventually, death. Researchers currently believe that aluminum toxicity (from the dialysate) contributes to the development of dialysis dementia.

Evaluation

A variety of laboratory tests will reveal the fact and extent of kidney failure; the simplest of these is an elevation of blood urea nitrogen (BUN). Abdominal X-ray will generally reveal the fact of small kidney size.

Outcome

Untreated, severe kidney failure leads rapidly to death. Dialysis can for many years sustain patients, who then suffer the obvious emotional drawback of depending for life upon a machine. There is also the threat of the complications mentioned earlier. A successful kidney transplant (cadaver or live donor) can reverse nearly all of these symptoms and relieve patients of the necessity of repeated dialyses.

KLINEFELTER'S SYNDROME

Occurrence	Age of onset	Gender	Refer to
Frequent	Birth	All male	Endocrinologist
What: Genetic male who has at least 47 chromosomes, including one Y and *two* X			
Physical: Tall; disproportionately long legs, small genitals, gynecomastia			
Mental: Mild mental retardation, criminal behavior, depression, psychosis			

At conception, children inherit 46 chromosomes comprising 23 pairs; one chromosome in each pair comes from each parent. Two of these 46 are sex chromosomes: From the mother, each person receives an X sex chromosome; the father may contribute either another X, in which case the child will be a girl, or a Y, which results in a boy baby.

But what if, through some mischance, a fetus receives a Y chromosome *and* two X's, for a total of 47? In humans (though not in all animals), it is the presence of a Y chromosome that determines maleness, so this 47-chromosome fetus will be a male. The individuals that result are termed Klinefelter males (guess the name of the person who first described the condition), and they present with some distinctive pathology.

This situation, with its many variants (e.g., XXXY), happens more often than you might think. Considering all genotypes, about 1 in 500 male babies is affected; Klinefelter's syndrome is a bit more common than Down's syndrome.

Physical Symptoms

As children, these boys don't look much different than their playmates, but with adolescence they grow taller than most men. Their height results from a lower body half that is long in proportion to the upper half. There may be fusion of the radius and ulna, the two bones of the forearm, so that they have difficulty rotating it.

Klinefelter males have small, firm testes that produce less testosterone than normal. As a result, their secondary sex characteristics remain underdeveloped: the penis is small; they have little body hair; they are troubled by infertility. They tend to have enlarged breasts (gynecomastia), and the risk of breast cancer, while still only about 20% of a woman's risk, is greatly increased. These men tend to be obese and to have varicose veins; some have diabetes mellitus, and there may be thyroid abnormalities as well. When present, acne may be severe.

Mental Symptoms

These patients have been reported to have a variety of other mental problems including depression, psychosis, low sexual activity, and, in seeming paradox, paraphilia. Fire-setting and other aggressive behaviors may be more common in Klinefelter males.

If the patient has two or more extra chromosomes, mental symptoms may be more likely or more severe. For example, XXYY patients may be borderline to mildly mentally retarded. An excess of criminal behavior and overrepresentation in prison populations has been reported among XXYY and XXXY patients.

Evaluation

Chromosome studies are definitive.

Outlook

Testosterone may ameliorate some of the effects of Klinefelter's syndrome, including, according to some reports, a reduction in fire-setting and other antisocial behaviors. Even without treatment, at least one follow-up study reveals that many of these patients manage to lead productive lives.

Special Note on Turner Females

Women can have sex chromosome abnormalities, too. When they do, there is far less to interest the mental health professional. About 1 in 2,000 girl babies is born with a single X chromosome. Genetically, these are "XO females." They have a number of physical defects: webbed neck, remarkably short stature (less than 5 feet tall), small jaw, and low-set ears. Although their external genitalia are normal, they have no internal sex organs. Of course, these women do not develop secondary sex characteristics, menstruate, or have children.

But few mental problems have been ascribed to the Turner female. The few studies reported find mild cognitive difficulties, such as problems discerning spatial relationships and handling numbers, but no serious cognitive difficulties such as mental retardation or dementia. Not surprisingly, considering their infertility and somewhat unusual appearance, these women may have social problems such as low self-esteem and lack of friends.

LIVER FAILURE

Occurrence	Age of onset	Gender	Refer to
Common	Increases with age	Males predominate	Gastroenterologist

What: Inability of liver to clear metabolic waste from the bloodstream

Physical: Jaundice, weakness, fatigue, anorexia, red palms, spider angiomas, easy bruising, tremor, motor incoordination

Mental: Irritability, depression, delirium

Unless it's smothered in onions on a plate, you probably don't think much about the liver. But it is the largest internal organ of the body (the skin weighs more, but it's outside!) and, with the kidneys, performs the vital function of removing toxic substances from the blood.

Overall, alcoholism is the most common cause of liver disease, and alcoholic liver disease is one of the five leading causes of death in the United States. But there are many other causes of liver disease besides drinking too much. For example, every year there are stories of people who have become seriously ill from eating shellfish contaminated by sewage. Infected by a virus called hepatitis B, these patients often go on to die or to suffer from chronic liver disease. Other causes include inherited conditions, Wilson's disease, and autoimmune disease.

Hepatitis and cirrhosis are by far the two most common manifestations of severe liver disease. Hepatitis is an inflammation of the liver that is usually the work of infection, but it also has other causes, including the use of certain medications (e.g., the popular painkiller, acetaminophen). The word cirrhosis means "scarring," and the liver becomes scarred as the result of prolonged liver disease. Hepatitis is one such cause, but most cirrhosis is caused by alcohol intake that is both prolonged (many years) and heavy (a pint per day or more of hard liquor). Hepatitis and cirrhosis have many symptoms in common.

Actually, we are born with far more liver than we need; it can perform its job adequately when functioning at only a fraction of its normal capacity. That's why so many patients with cirrhosis don't show much in the way of symptoms for many years. Even a patient whose liver has been nearly destroyed by chronic alcohol intake may have few mental symptoms. It is important to recognize such patients, however, because they are so much at risk for even more serious problems.

Physical Symptoms

Acute viral hepatitis usually begins abruptly with nausea, lack of appetite and, in smokers, a characteristic distaste for tobacco smoke. Many patients develop fever as well as abdominal pain and liver tenderness (under the lower right rib cage). As the liver becomes unable to do its job, jaundice (yellow skin) develops, and the patient's stools become nearly white in color (the usual brown color is due to excreted bilirubin).

As the disease becomes chronic, other symptoms appear. These include painful joints, absent menses, acne, increased body hair, obesity, and Cushing's syndrome (q.v.). In addition, there can appear skin symptoms, as described later for cirrhosis.

The palms of the hands of cirrhosis patients typically develop a chronic ruddiness (palmar erythema), best seen along the fleshy part that extends from the fifth finger to the wrist. Normally tiny blood vessels on the upper trunk, face, and upper arms become enlarged; from a central point, they send out short, crooked extensions that resemble the spokes of a wheel (spider angiomas). This typical appearance inspired a nursery rhyme parody that has been learned by generations of pathology students:

> A modern Miss Muffet decided to rough it
> And live upon whiskey and gin.
> Red hands and a spider developed outside her—
> Such is the wages of sin.

Cirrhosis patients may bruise very easily, and with increasing malnutrition, they become weak and fatigued. Men lose body hair and gain breast mass (gynecomastia); women may have increased body hair (hirsuitism) and complain of menstrual irregularities. With advanced cirrhosis, the liver is unable to eliminate bilirubin, the breakdown product of old red blood cells, producing the characteristic jaundice.

In biliary cirrhosis, drinking is not the cause, but then, no one knows what the cause is (a disordered immune response has been suggested, of course). This form is found predominantly in women, for whom itching is a prominent early symptom; this may be generalized or confined in its early stages to the palms of the hands and soles of the feet.

Once liver disease progresses far enough for hepatic encephalopathy to develop, tremor and motor incoordination may occur. The patient's breath takes on a musty smell (fetor hepaticus).

Perhaps the most characteristic (at least, most classical) physical indication of encephalopathy is a flapping motion of the hand at the wrist, seen when patients hold their arms up with palms facing outward as if to signal "stop." This flapping motion is called asterixis. Motor incoordination may produce difficulty walking. The neurological symptoms may fluctuate with time.

Mental Symptoms

Up to the point that encephalopathy develops, there may be no noticeable changes in the patient's mental state. (Typical alcohol-related dementia and delirium are due to more direct effects of toxins or malnutrition on the brain, rather than being mediated through liver disease.) However, some patients with acute hepatitis note temporary irritability or difficulties with concentration. In chronic hepatitis, low mood and fatigue may suggest depressive disease.

When most of the liver has been destroyed, blood coming from the intestines no longer flows through the liver at all. This allows toxic products, such as ammonia, clear sailing from the intestines to the brain. Then, the most common mental manifestation of chronic liver disease, hepatic encephalopathy, becomes evident.

Encephalopathy usually begins slowly. The patient becomes mentally dull and drowsy, frequently yawning and even napping inappropriately. There may be the problems with focusing attention and other evidence of impaired thinking typical of delirium. Mood changes (especially irritability and labile affect) may also be noted. In the later stages, more extensive deterioration in self-care may be noted, and eventually stupor and even coma develop.

Evaluation

Depending on the severity of impairment, liver enzymes will be elevated, and there may be anemia. In jaundiced patients, serum bilirubin will be elevated. Most patients who have hepatic encephalopathy will have an elevated serum ammonia level.

Outcome

Because it destroys less tissue, hepatitis is usually less lethal than cirrhosis. But too often, drinking continues, and the patient goes on to develop cirrhosis, then encephalopathy.

Mental symptoms should resolve once the underlying condition has been corrected. Too often, this does not happen—hepatitis becomes chronic or the alcoholic patient begins drinking again. Medical treatment can improve even hepatic encephalopathy, but for some, liver transplantation may be the only hope.

LYME DISEASE

Occurrence	Age of onset	Gender	Refer to
Frequent	All ages	About equal	Internist
What: Infectious disease transmitted by bite of a tiny tick			
Physical: Headache, fever, chills, pains, fatigue, malaise, stiff neck, paralysis, arthritis			
Mental: Depression, psychosis, anxiety, mild cognitive symptoms			

Lyme disease, properly known as Lyme borreliosis, is the most recently identified disorder covered in this book. Yet, it is far from rare—over 1,000 cases per year are reported in this country alone, and it is also endemic throughout much of Europe.

Named for the picturesque town in Connecticut where it was recognized in 1975, Lyme disease is caused by a microorganism belonging to the same family that causes syphilis. This spirochete, *Borrelia burgdorferi*, is transmitted by a tick so small that most people don't even remember being bitten. The tick is carried by mice and deer, especially those indigenous to Wisconsin, Minnesota, and the Northeast, from Maryland to Massachusetts. Hikers, campers, and other outdoors people are especially at risk for contracting this disease, which, not surprisingly, is most often reported during the summer months.

B. burgdorferi is an equal-opportunity infectious agent, affecting all ages and both sexes.

Physical Symptoms

Laboratory texts note that *B. burgdorferi* grows best on a complex culture medium, but it thrives nicely in humans, too. The skin lesion begins as a small, red dot that may be raised; it expands to form a larger, round lesion. (Because it grows and moves, this pattern is called erythema migrans.) Several days later, the patient develops a flu-like illness, with headache, fever, chills, and pains that seem to move from one muscle or joint to another. These symptoms wax and wane in intensity, but the fatigue and sick feeling (malaise) tend to persist.

Weeks to months later, about 15% of those who have not been adequately treated will develop neurological symptoms such as paralysis of facial muscles, meningitis (stiff neck), or encephalitis. A few patients develop heart block, which is often asymptomatic but can cause palpitations, dizziness, and even loss of consciousness. Still later, if still not treated, over half will develop the painful, swollen joints of full-blown arthritis.

Mental Symptoms

Various reports suggest that anywhere from one-fourth to two-thirds of patients will have symptoms of depression, which may not necessarily fulfill criteria for a major depressive episode. Undoubtedly, the fatigue and difficulty sleeping typical of Lyme disease contribute to the diagnosis of depression.

Many patients develop a mild encephalopathy—they show some difficulty remembering things and some loss of mental flexibility. Psychotic symptoms suggesting a schizophreniform or paranoid psychosis have also been reported. Anxiety symptoms, including panic attacks and even obsessive–compulsive behavior, have also been reported. Some patients have been noted to develop symptoms of anorexia nervosa.

Evaluation

A serum antibody response develops to *B. burgdorferi,* but false negatives are possible. Suspect Lyme disease in anyone with atypical mental symptoms, who lives in an area endemic for the disease or has a history of tick bite or erythema migrans.

Outlook

Most patients recover completely with a course of oral antibiotics, which may also eliminate psychotic and depressive symptoms. However, complete resolution of all symptoms may take months or even longer, and several weeks of antibiotics of treatment—or repeated courses of treatment—may be necessary. After months or years untreated, the arthritis may become chronic. If the tick is removed intact within 24 hours, infection by the spirochete may be prevented.

MÉNIÈRE'S SYNDROME

Occurrence	Age of onset	Gender	Refer to
Frequent	40–50	Males predominate	Neurologist
What: Neurological disorder of unknown cause			
Physical: Dizziness with nausea and vomiting, tinnitus, nystagmus, eventual deafness			
Mental: Anxiety, panic attacks, difficulty concentrating, depression			

Do you remember, as a child, the wonderful giddy sensation you felt from spinning around on skates until you were so dizzy you could hardly stand? Ménière's syndrome is a bit like that, except that you don't need skates, and it isn't wonderful. It is a peculiar neurological disorder in which, sometimes with astonishing suddenness, the patient becomes acutely dizzy. There's also ringing in the ears and deafness, but these symptoms come later.

Ménière's is also not a disorder of childhood—it doesn't usually affect patients until they reach their 40s. Although not exactly common, it is not rare. One or two people per 10,000 are diagnosed, men two or three times more often than women.

Physical Symptoms

In all mammals, humans being no exception, the organ of balance is located in intimate association with the inner ear. It should therefore come as no surprise that the episodes of dizziness are associated with ringing in the ears (tinnitus). This ringing is experienced as a low-pitched buzz, worse during the attacks of dizziness, but usually persisting between episodes. As the disease continues over months and years, there is hearing loss, which may worsen until the patient becomes deaf in the affected ear. The attacks themselves may last only a few minutes or as long as several hours. In two-thirds of the cases, the ringing and deafness occur unilaterally.

The episodes of dizziness are often accompanied by nausea, vomiting, and heavy sweating; nystagmus (rapid oscillation of the eyeball, usually back and forth, but sometimes up and down) is experienced during attacks also. A very few patients may actually lose consciousness. The attacks themselves occur sporadically and unpredictably—weeks or months may go by between episodes. If left untreated, they may increase in frequency until they occur almost daily.

Mental Symptoms

When the illness is mild and dizziness is experienced more as a slight instability or fullness in the head, patients may be misdiagnosed as having an anxiety or mood disorder. Symptoms compatible with major depressive disorder have been reported in patients with Ménière's. Panic attacks have also been reported.

Evaluation

No one really knows what causes Ménière's syndrome. Swelling of a part of the balancing mechanism of the inner ear has been suspected for generations but remains unproven. Virtually alone, of all the physical disorders discussed in this book, Ménière's syndrome has no available laboratory tests. The diagnosis is made solely on clinical grounds. But testing (X-ray, serum glucose) is vital to exclude acoustic nerve tumor and diabetic neuropathy, which can mimic the symptoms of Ménière's.

Outlook

There is also no specific treatment; bed rest is the most effective management for an acute episode. Sometimes, after years of recurrent attacks, the syndrome simply disappears.

MENOPAUSE

Occurrence	Age of onset	Gender	Refer to
Normal	40s–50s	Females	Gynecologist
What: Hormonal changes that occur in women in their 40s or 50s			
Physical: Hot flashes, decreased breast mass, vaginal dryness			
Mental: Irritability, depression, insomnia, anxiety, forgetfulness			

If most adults don't think much about menopause, it is probably because they are either men and will never go through it or women under the age of 50, who haven't yet had the experience. But I have it on good authority that women in the throes think about menopause quite a bit. Menopause can hardly be called a disease in the sense that it is a normal event in the life of any middle-aged women and many not so middle-aged—it is surgically induced in about one-third of women in the United States. But in the sense that it often produces symptoms that require medical attention, menopause is a physiological state that should be taken seriously by all healthcare practitioners.

Physical Symptoms

Several symptoms can affect how a woman feels, and how she feels about herself. Loss of bone calcium can lead to fractures, especially of the hip and spine. Vaginal dryness and loss of breast mass can affect her self-image. But the problem that causes the most mischief by far is hot flashes.

The hot flash (or hot flush; at night it is sometimes called night sweats) is a nearly universal symptom of menopause that is annoying in its own right and can lead to additional mental symptoms. It typically begins with a sense of warmth of the head and face. This gives rise to facial flushing that spreads rapidly across the neck and to other parts of the body. The pulse rate increases. The woman feels hot and may perspire heavily. The need for cooling may cause her to fan herself or to throw off the bedclothes. An entire episode may last 3 minutes or so and can recur as often as every hour.

Mental Symptoms

Hot flashes at night interfere with sleep, but there are other disorders of sleep that accompany menopause: an increase in the time it takes to get to sleep (latency) and a decrease in the amount of REM sleep. As a consequence, the patient feels unrested. Other psychological symptoms are likely to occur, especially just before the menses stop (in nonsurgical cases). These include irritability and a sense of anxiety. Some women may complain of forgetfulness or have trouble concentrating; others feel depressed.

Evaluation

A low serum estrogen level or elevated follicle stimulating hormone level will only confirm that which, in most cases, should be obvious to any layperson. Testing hormone levels may be useful in patients who begin to have symptoms in their 30s or early 40s.

Outcome

Although symptoms can persist for 5 years or sometimes longer, menopause is a self-limiting condition. Despite the (now discarded) concept of involutional melancholia, menopause is not causally associated with any serious mental disorders.

MIGRAINE

Occurrence	Age of onset	Gender	Refer to
Common	Puberty	Females predominate	Neurologist
What: Familial neurological syndrome of unknown cause			
Physical: Severe unilateral headache, photo- and phonophobia, nausea			
Mental: Lethargy, irritability, anxiety symptoms, depression			

On the road to Damascus, Saul of Tarsus was beset by a bright, flashing light that caused him to fall to the ground. Various scholars have suggested that this was due to a seizure or eye pathology, but at least one latter-day writer believes that Saul's attack and subsequent "thorn in the Flesh" was actually caused by migraine. The name, which dates to the Middle Ages, is a corruption of the ancient term hemicrania (literally, "half-head"), referring to the tendency of this type of headache to be one-sided.

Whatever beset Saul, throughout the ages, migraine has presented its sufferers with a significant cross to bear. Migraine is not just a bad headache, but a constellation of neurological symptoms that cause patients to feel terribly ill and, at their worst, totally incapacitated for any mental or physical activity. It is apparently mediated by the neurotransmitter serotonin.

There is a strong hereditary presumption in this common affliction, but no one knows exactly what causes the symptoms themselves. They used to be considered vascular, but more recent theories hold that they are primarily neuronal. Attacks can be triggered by a wide variety of precipitants—hunger, alcohol, stress and mental tension, fatigue, bright lights, and foods that contain the substance tyramine (aged cheese, such as cheddar or Swiss, is the most common of these).

Migraine attacks commonly begin around the time of puberty. There is no known racial predisposition for this common, distressing, yet benign condition that affects around 10% of adults. Women are afflicted about twice as frequently as men and often will have attacks during the few days before their menstrual periods. For reasons that are unclear, a woman's migraine symptoms often disappear during pregnancy.

Physical Symptoms

Four out of five sufferers (they are sometimes called migraineures) have what is called common migraine, or migraine without aura. This just means that nothing special happens that tells the patient that a migraine is on its way. Typically, migraine headaches are one-sided and pulsating; they are made worse by light, sound, smells, or physical activity. The patient feels nauseated and may even vomit, and will retreat to bed in a darkened room, utterly unable to pursue ordinary activities for as brief a time as 4 hours and as long as 3 days. Some patients may sweat excessively, have trouble speaking clearly, or complain of water retention that can produce swelling of extremities. Some may have severe neck, shoulder, or even abdominal pain, without necessarily experiencing the headache; these attacks are known as migraine equivalents.

The 10% or so of patients who do have an aura (classical migraine) experience it principally as one-sided visual changes. This may be a blind spot that begins centrally and gradually expands outward in an arc, accompanied by flashing lights (scintillating scotoma). One patient described it as looking like a diamond-back rattlesnake that gradually slithered to the visual periphery. Other premonitory symptoms may include weakness, aphasia, and numbness or tingling of the extremities, but almost always there are visual symptoms as well.

Mental Symptoms

During an attack, patients are irritable and moody and, like Garbo, want only "to be left alone." They may also complain of slowed thinking. Rarely, a patient will complain of visual illusions (e.g., a dead relative) that might be mistakenly ascribed to psychosis. Migraine headaches have been associated with major depression and even with bipolar mood disorders, though the exact relationship remains to be worked out.

Evaluation

There are no laboratory tests that reliably distinguish migraine phenomena from other types of headache or from other illnesses, for that matter. Usually, the history and family history are definitive.

Outcome

Of course, for most people, migraine does not often have as profound an effect as it did for Saul, who, subsequent to his experience, became the Apostle Paul. But though migraine can have a devastating effect on a patient's quality of life, it is benign in terms of life expectancy. Intensity of attacks and severity of headache may abate after menopause. Many excellent strategies for treatment and prevention are available, including several recently introduced medications. In fact, of all the chronic disorders mentioned in this book, the treatment of migraine has seen the most substantial recent advances.

Note on Tension Headache

Most headaches, of course, are not of the migraine variety at all but are caused by something else. Usually, they are referred to as tension headaches, with the presumption that they are caused by muscle contraction at the front or back of the skull. No one knows whether they have anything to do with stress or mental tension. They occur more often in women, tend to be bilateral, are not generally worsened by physical activity, and are unaccompanied by nausea, vomiting, or the need to avoid light or sound.

MITRAL VALVE PROLAPSE

Occurrence	Age of onset	Gender	Refer to
Common	Especially 14–30	Females predominate	Cardiologist
What: "Floppy" heart valve allows reflux of blood back into lungs			
Physical: Usually none; chest pain, palpitations, breathlessness, fainting			
Mental: Panic attacks			

Mitral valve prolapse (MVP) syndrome has had a checkered history. Within the last few decades it has been discovered, proclaimed as a major cause of panic disorder, recognized as occurring (albeit in diverse degrees) in up to 20% of the general population, and now, finally, cast aside by some clinicians as having little clinical relevance. For better or for worse, then, here are the facts.

The heart performs two important circulatory functions. It pumps venous (oxygen-depleted) blood through the lungs, then back to the heart; it then pumps the newly oxygenated blood throughout the rest of the body for use by its cells. The function of the mitral valve is to prevent oxygenated blood from being pumped backward to the lungs when the heart beats.

Some people are born with a mitral valve whose leaflets are too relaxed. These "floppy" valves allow some blood to leak backward with each heartbeat. This causes a murmur and a clicking sound that can be heard with a stethoscope. Although these floppy valves are physically thickened, most patients are asymptomatic and live a normal life span, completely unaware that they have MVP.

Physical Symptoms

Associated with more serious degrees of MVP are chest pain with palpitations and rapid heartbeat, shortness of breath, tiredness, fainting, and lightheadedness.

Mental Symptoms

Many of these people have what appear to be classical panic attacks, and the entire MVP syndrome has been reported to be more common in patients who have panic disorder. But recent reports suggest that there is little, if any, difference between panic disorder with and without MVP. It also appears that antipanic drugs work equally well in the two sets of patients. The conclusion: In the world of anxiety symptoms, MVP may represent a distinction without a difference.

Evaluation

A test called an echocardiogram has the best chance of detecting any physical abnormality.

Outlook

The current consensus holds that panic attacks are panic attacks, with or without MVP, which therefore has little clinical relevance. Even so, patients with severe symptoms of panic attack should probably be referred to a cardiologist for evaluation. Most will need no other medical treatment than simple reassurance. For the most severely affected, symptoms may progress over years or decades unless antipanic medications are employed.

MULTIPLE SCLEROSIS

Occurrence	Age of onset	Gender	Refer to
Frequent	20–40	Females predominate	Neurologist
What: Loss of myelin sheath in patches throughout the central nervous system			
Physical: Weakness, visual problems, incontinence, trouble walking, fatigue, paresthesias			
Mental: Depression, mania, sudden emotionality, cognitive impairment, dementia			

At least in the United States, where it affects more than 1 person in 1,000 in the general population, multiple sclerosis (MS) is frequently encountered. But one of the mysteries of this neurological affliction is that it is uncommon among Japanese and almost unheard of in Black Africans. There may be an inherited tendency to develop the disease (siblings of MS patients have a lifetime risk of around 3%; for identical twins, it is around 30%), but the underlying cause has not been determined. Both immunological and viral etiologies have had their champions.

Myelin is the substance that composes the sheath that surrounds each nerve in the central nervous system (CNS) as well as the peripheral nerves. In MS, for reasons that are unclear, there is patchy loss of myelin from various areas of the brain and spinal cord. When that happens, the neurons are no longer protected and cannot function. They are replaced by scar tissue (sclerosis) that is called plaque.

As to the effect of geography upon incidence of MS, no one has ever offered a completely satisfactory explanation. But it is now well established that the farther you live from the equator, the more likely you are to develop this disorder. Furthermore, this tendency appears to become fixed by about the age of 15. Children born near the equator who move to higher incidence areas prior to puberty will have the greater chance of developing the disorder. Whatever the etiology of MS, somehow the environment in which the individual was reared plays a causative role. To minimize your risk of developing this relatively common and often heartbreaking disease, be sure that you were reared in a tropical climate.

Physical Symptoms

Because plaques can occur nearly anywhere in the CNS, the symptoms of MS vary widely. Prominent among them is muscle weakness, especially of the limbs (difficulty climbing stairs), lower face, and eye (double vision, blurred vision). Other visual symptoms include diminished acuity, blind spots, and even loss of color perception. Genitourinary symptoms can include incontinence and erectile impotence. Some patients become so uncoordinated as to have difficulty walking (ataxia). Others complain of paresthesias (numbness or tingling of extremities), fatigue, trouble speaking, and many, many other physical problems. Some symptoms are so bizarre as to defy understanding—such as trouble recognizing faces in the absence of demonstrable CNS lesions. With such varying symptoms, it is no wonder that MS patients are sometimes dismissed as having hysteria.

Mental Symptoms

These can be discussed under four headings.

Mania

The classical picture of MS, the one described in so many medical school neurology lectures, is of euphoria that is unreasonable in the light of such serious physical symptoms. The affect of such individuals is sometimes described as *la belle indifférence* (French for "lofty indifference"). This seeming indifference to the seriousness of illness may come from damage to the frontal lobes, but it is also sometimes encountered in patients with somatization disorder. Although true bipolar mood disorder is probably overrepresented by up to twofold in populations of MS patients, mania is far from being the dominant affect. Nonetheless, up to 25% of MS patients may be inappropriately euphoric at some time during their illness.

Depression

Rather, many MS patients (in some series, half or more) are depressed. No wonder, you might think, considering the amount of disability they face relatively early in their lives. But depression is more likely in MS patients than in those with other serious medical illnesses, suggesting something physiological about the cause–effect relationship. Therefore, even though many such patients may meet the criteria for major depressive episode, the appropriate diagnosis would usually be depressive disorder due to MS.

Emotional Incontinence

This refers to the sudden onset of laughing or (especially) weeping without an appropriate precipitant.

Cognitive Impairment

To some degree or other, problems with thinking and memory probably occur in half or more of MS patients. Especially during the earlier phases of the disorder, there may be only a mild loss of memory, but more clinically important, dementia can also occur. Judgment may be impaired, and the patient may have difficulty forming new memories.

Evaluation

MRI will often show multiple areas of plaque within the substance of the brain.

Outlook

Because of its variability, the course of this illness can be another source of confusion. Symptoms usually begin suddenly and last for several weeks. Then, they will typically fade away, not to reappear for perhaps months or years. Patients often have residual disability between attacks of the disease, but sometimes they seem to return completely to normal. But more usually, over many years, disability gradually accumulates with repeated attacks, though the degree is highly variable.

Nearly half of all patients have a relatively benign course, with little or no disability. After 25 years, half the patients in one sample were still ambulatory, and one-fourth were still working.

MYASTHENIA GRAVIS

Occurrence	Age of onset	Gender	Refer to
Frequent	See text	Females predominate	Neurologist
What: Autoimmune disorder of neuromuscular transmission			
Physical: Muscle weakness			
Mental: Anxiety, minor cognitive symptoms, memory loss			

The name of this disease literally means "severely weak muscles," which describes perfectly the major symptom. These patients, typically young women, may be unable to hold their eyes fully open, to chew their food thoroughly, or to climb more than a few stairs at a time. When you consider that these rather bizarre symptoms can come and go, sometimes within the space of a few minutes, it is no wonder that these patients are sometimes misdiagnosed as having hysteria or other primary mental disorders.

But myasthenia gravis is a disorder of neuromuscular transmission. Normally, the neurotransmitter acetylcholine carries the message from the nerve to the muscle, telling it to contract. When an autoimmune mechanism destroys many of the receptor sites on the muscle for acetylcholine, fewer impulses get through, and the muscle cannot work as hard as it needs to. The result is rapid fatigue of affected muscles, without the sense of being tired.

Affecting about 1 in 10,000 people, myasthenia gravis is not rare. But it does have an unusual pattern of distribution. When it affects younger adults (ages 20–40), as is usually the case, three-fourths of the patients are women. But in the 50–70 age group, patients are more likely to be men.

Physical Symptoms

Of course, there is muscle weakness, and it is often profound. And the degree of the patient's strength can vary from month to month, week to week, and even hour to hour. Patients often note that sleep temporarily restores strength. The pattern of muscle involvement in myasthenia gravis is also distinctive. Muscles of the eyes and face are almost always involved. Early symptoms often include double vision and an inability to keep the eyelids more than half-open. Smiles become crooked, and chewing and swallowing are a chore. Later, the extremities usually become involved, especially the thighs and upper arms. Even breathing can be affected, rendering patients vulnerable to pneumonia. Complicating the diagnostic picture is the fact that these patients often have other diseases of autoimmune origin, such as thyroid disease, rheumatoid arthritis, or systemic lupus erythematosus.

Mental Symptoms

Although they readily admit their muscle weakness, myasthenia patients do not especially note that they are tired in the sense of feeling weary. They may complain of anxiety symptoms, especially if they are having difficulty breathing. They may have cognitive problems (such as with memory) as well—several recent studies have found that myasthenia patients score less well than matched controls on the MMSE.

Evaluation

Edrophonium (Tensilon) is a drug that will very briefly inhibit the enzyme that deactivates acetylcholine. Hence, the Tensilon test: An intravenous injection of the drug dramatically and almost instantly improves strength in the affected muscles. The effect lasts only a few minutes, just long enough to confirm the diagnosis.

Outlook

For reasons that after decades of experience are still not understood, removal of the thymus gland, which is located in the front part of the upper chest, just above the heart, usually produces dramatic improvement in the patient's strength. Although improvement may be delayed by many months, sometimes there is a downright cure. Drugs are also useful, so that nearly all patients, 25% of whom used to succumb to respiratory infection, can look forward to a normal, useful life span.

NEUROCUTANEOUS DISORDERS

Occurrence	Age of onset	Gender	Refer to
Frequent	Any age	About equal	Neurologist
What: Often inherited (dominant), nonmalignant tumors of nerve and skin			
Physical: Seizure disorders, obvious skin pathology			
Mental: Mental retardation, depression, anxiety, dementia			

This term covers several conditions that we don't often think much about, but that nonetheless affect sizable numbers of adults and children. As the name suggests, the symptoms of neurocutaneous disorders affect nerves and skin. The pathology is primarily due to tumors that, though usually not malignant, cause mischief by their location in the brain and other parts of the nervous system and misery because of the unsightly appearance of the skin. I'll modify the usual structure to cover these several conditions in separate parts of this section. They are all inherited as dominant genes, and each can be associated with mental retardation.

Neurofibromatosis

Also called von Recklinghausen disease, neurofibromatosis is the most common of these disorders; it affects around 1 person in 5,000. When tumors affect the peripheral nerves, they appear as small (up to 5 cm or so) nodules under the skin that can become pedunculated (attached by a stalk). A patient may have thousands of these growths on the torso and extremities. When neurofibromas grow in the brain, sensory and motor symptoms may be present (deafness occurs when such a tumor grows on the acoustic nerve). Those located on the arms, legs, and body generally cause few problems other than cosmetic ones.

These patients also have brownish areas up to several centimeters across that are called *café au lait,* or coffee with cream, spots. (For a person to have just a few of them is perfectly normal—you can see at least two such spots on Sharon Stone in the movie *Casino.*)

Malformations within the CNS, which is often a complication of neurofibromatosis, can yield a variety of mental disorders. As many as one-third of patients have a mild degree of mental retardation; depressive and anxiety disorders may affect another third.

For many years, neurofibromatosis was thought responsible for the grotesque appearance of Joseph Merrick, who in Victorian England was known as the Elephant Man. That this disorder has been called Elephant Man's disease is rendered somewhat ironic by a recent reanalysis of Merrick's bones. The new study revealed that he actually suffered from a rare condition now known as Proteus syndrome, which is not hereditary at all, rather than neurofibromatosis. Proteus syndrome is caused by malfunctioning cellular growth.

Tuberous Sclerosis

Less common, but more devastating, tuberous sclerosis affects around 1 in 15,000 persons. As with neurofibromatosis, the skin lesions are the least troubling manifestation. They first appear in early childhood as small, red pinheads dusted across the nose and both cheeks. As the child ages they enlarge, eventually becoming shiny, yellow sebaceous adenomas.

Although hard, fibrous nodules resembling potatoes (hence the name) may appear in many other sites, such as liver, kidney, retina, those that occur in the brain are the most problematic. They are firm, white nodules that vary in size and take up space that should be occupied by brain tissue. The result is mental retardation in around two-thirds of patients and seizures in most. Diagnosis is confirmed by skull X-rays and CT scan.

Although some patients who have only skin lesions may be relatively unaffected, those with CNS involvement may have a progressive dementia. Autism has also been reported in some patients with tuberous sclerosis.

Sturge–Weber Disease

Actually, this disease is rarely hereditary (geneticists would say that it occurs sporadically). Although no one really knows what causes it, the manifestations are well defined. These patients have a dark, red patch on one side of the face, called a port-wine stain, with a tumor of the blood vessels inside the skull. This tumor causes progressive loss of adjacent brain tissue, which, in turn, leads to seizures, paralysis of the opposite side of the body, and glaucoma. Although many patients have developmental delay and often severe mental retardation, one-third or more are able to be financially self-sufficient. Diagnosis can be made by visualizing calcium deposits within the brain, which can be seen even by conventional X-ray.

Mikhail Gorbachev has a port-wine stain, but to my knowledge he, like most people who have them, doesn't have Sturge–Weber disease.

NORMAL PRESSURE HYDROCEPHALUS

Occurrence	Age of onset	Gender	Refer to
See text	Any age	About equal	Neurologist
What: Fluid collects inside the brain, dilating ventricles and squeezing brain tissue			
Physical: Trouble walking, urinary incontinence, headache, weakness			
Mental: Dementia, mood swings, psychosis			

Hydrocephalus means "water on the brain." Of course, it isn't literally *on* the brain, but rather inside it, and it isn't water but cerebrospinal fluid (CSF). CSF is manufactured deep inside cavities of the brain, known as ventricles. It normally flows toward the spinal cord through several small apertures, called the aqueducts. If these small openings become even partly blocked, fluid collects inside the ventricles, causing them to expand without an increase in CSF pressure, hence the name.

The mere fact that there is excess fluid is not the problem, rather it is that the skull is a rigid box containing a nonexpandable amount of space. The more room the fluid occupies, the less room there is for brain tissue. It is the gradual squeezing, and eventual death, of brain tissue that causes symptoms to develop.

Exact data are not usually given, but normal pressure hydrocephalus (NPH) is not a common condition. (Congenital hydrocephalus, caused by malformation during fetal development, is encountered in about 1 in every 500 births, but it is not relevant to this discussion.) Although hydrocephalus in adults can result from head injury or infectious diseases, usually the underlying cause is unknown. Hydrocephalus can affect adults of any age.

Physical Symptoms

Difficulty walking (ataxia) is characteristic of this disorder; in this case, a slow gait with the feet planted wide apart is especially typical. Urinary incontinence is found in perhaps half the patients. The three symptoms—ataxia, incontinence, and dementia—constitute the classic triad associated with NPH, though most patients will not have all three of these symptoms. Headache, weakness, and malaise (feeling sick) have also been noted.

Mental Symptoms

When mental symptoms are present, they are usually cognitive. Intellectual deterioration, with a reduced level of awareness, begins insidiously and progresses gradually over a period of many weeks or months. Memory loss can range from mild to profound. There have been reports of mood swings in a few patients, some of whom improved once surgical shunting led to reduced ventricular size. Psychosis (delusions or hallucinations) has been reported only rarely and is at times associated with catatonia or violent behavior.

Evaluation

MRI or CT scan of the head will demonstrate enlarged ventricles of the brain.

Outcome

As with most other disorders, the prognosis depends upon a variety of factors, including age of the patient, duration of illness, the presence of other medical diseases, and whether they are causative or merely associated with NPH. However, neuro-surgical shunting procedures, in which CSF is continuously drained from within the brain, lead to improvement in around half of these patients. All too often, the diagnosis is not made until it is too late for the patient to recover substantially from the intellectual deterioration.

ally become demented, far more than is true of the general population.

The use of even small amounts of medication in demented parkinsonism patients can produce the side effect of delirium (vivid dreams or insomnia progressing to delusions, visual hallucinations, and agitation).

Special Note on Causation

Among mental health patients, perhaps the most common cause of Parkinson-like symptoms are the neuroleptic drugs (such as chlorpromazine, fluphenazine, haloperidol) that have been used since the mid-1950s to treat psychosis. Although many symptoms of this drug-induced pseudoparkinsonism can be managed with careful reduction of the medicine or the use of antiparkinsonian medications, tremor, loss of facial mobility, and shuffling gait remain common among mental health patients who require continuing use of neuroleptic medication. Another, less common cause is from multiple blows to the head. This is what happened to Muhammad Ali, the poetic heavyweight boxer who once could "float like a butterfly, sting like a bee." Even rarer is a severe form of parkinsonism that has afflicted some young people after taking MPTP, an illegal opioid drug similar to meperidine.

Evaluation

The diagnosis is established by the presence of typical symptoms and physical examination.

Outlook

Once diagnosed, the progress of this disorder can be very variable, running anywhere from several years to decades, before death eventually ensues. Medications, extraordinarily helpful in managing symptoms, have even extended the life span of these patients. Physical disability can be delayed or, in some cases, prevented altogether by the patient's diligent adherence to a program of physical activity.

PELLAGRA

Occurrence	Age of onset	Gender	Refer to
Rare	Older persons	Males predominate	Internist
What: Symptoms caused by a dietary deficiency of niacin			
Physical: Weakness, anorexia, headache, diarrhea, skin red and rough			
Mental: Depression, anxiety, delirium, dementia			

Pellagra (pronounce it to rhyme with Niagara) is a chronic, wasting disease that is due to the deficiency of niacin, also known as nicotinic acid, a close relative of nicotine. It was formerly endemic in the southern part of the United States and is still found in developing countries where diets consist primarily of corn, which the rest of the world calls maize. With improved nutrition and education about vitamins, it has almost disappeared from Western countries. However, it is occasionally still encountered in the United States among patients who derive most of their calories from alcohol and in some sufferers from carcinoid syndrome (q.v.).

Physical Symptoms

For centuries, pellagra was considered primarily to be a disease of the skin. (The word comes from Latin and Greek roots meaning "rough skin.") The dermatitis occurs as a reaction to sunlight and may at first look like sunburn. It progresses to reddish-brown, scaly, roughened areas of skin, especially on the hands, wrists, knees, and feet. Mucus membranes are also involved, and the tongue may become shiny and beefy red in appearance. Down in the intestines, similar changes take place, and a severe, watery diarrhea results. Other early symptoms include weakness and loss of appetite. Headache and dizziness may also occur.

Mental Symptoms

Early on, these may simulate mood or anxiety disorders: irritability, fatigue, apathy, sleeplessness, depression, and anxiety. As the disease progresses, patients may become confused and completely disoriented, not even knowing who they are. Hallucinations may ensue; ultimately, dementia may set in. Three of the classic "4 D's" of pellagra are thus dermatitis, diarrhea, and dementia.

Evaluation

No laboratory tests are likely to aid in the diagnosis of this condition. Diagnosis depends on the characteristic history and symptoms. This is unfortunate, inasmuch as clinicians' suspicion will be extremely low due to the rarity of pellagra in Western countries.

Outlook

Vitamin therapy, or perhaps merely the resumption of an adequate diet, leads to rapid improvement of symptoms. Without treatment comes the fourth D of pellagra: death.

PERNICIOUS ANEMIA

Occurrence	Age of onset	Gender	Refer to
Common	60s or later	Equal	Hematologist
What: Deficiency of vitamin B$_{12}$ due to malabsorption from small intestine			
Physical: Anemia, dizziness, ringing in ears, palpitations, glossy tongue			
Mental: Personality change (irritability), forgetfulness, depression, dementia, psychosis			

Usually, when we think of anemia, we think of iron deficiency; the phrase "tired blood," once used to hawk an iron tonic, comes to mind. In any event, anemia is seldom associated with mental illness. But anemia is not a single disease, and pernicious anemia (PA) is notorious for causing serious mental symptoms.

PA is a deficiency of cobalamin (vitamin B_{12}). This vitamin is necessary in protein synthesis (it helps convert one amino acid, homocysteine, to another, methionine). We can't make it ourselves, and plants don't have it, so the only way we can get this vital substance is from meat or dairy products. With the help of intrinsic factor, which is produced by the lining of the stomach, dietary cobalamin is absorbed from the small intestine and then stored in the liver. The human body can store enough cobalamin to last several years, so you can see that the degree and duration of malabsorption must be pretty severe to cause symptoms.

Because animals provide the main source of vitamin B_{12}, you would imagine that strict vegetarians could have problems with PA—but they can take vitamin tablets. In fact, most PA patients are people who lack intrinsic factor and therefore cannot absorb cobalamin into the bloodstream. (Some authors reserve the PA diagnosis for *only* these patients.) Other patients develop the disease due to surgical removal of the stomach. It is thought that underlying PA may be an immunological abnormality, similar to hypothyroidism, hypoparathyroidism, and insulin-dependent diabetes mellitus.

The disease is much more common than you might think: Nearly 1% of Americans will have it at some time during their lifetime. Americans of Asian descent are less affected than are those of European or African background.

Physical Symptoms

PA develops gradually and progresses slowly, sometimes over a period of years. Of course there is anemia, with attendant weakness and fatigue. Other complaints may include dizziness and ringing in the ears (tinnitus). Because there are fewer oxygen-carrying red blood cells than normal, a patient's heart must pump hard and fast to supply the body's tissues with oxygen, hence, the sensation of palpitations. Some patients complain of sore tongue, which, on inspection, is glossy, smooth, and red. They may also have loss of appetite and other gastrointestinal symptoms, including diarrhea.

So far, the symptoms are generally reversible with effective treatment. But as the disease progresses, the nerve sheaths become affected in a process known as demyelination. With damage to their protective coverings, the nerves themselves begin to degenerate and will eventually die. Because nerves cannot regenerate, their loss is irreversible. The symptoms produced include weakness, numbness, trouble walking, and paresthesias (pins-and-needles sensations). Some patients will have trouble controlling bowels or bladder.

Mental Symptoms

The majority of PA patients will probably have some degree of mental symptoms, which in some cases are the first to develop. Some patients become only mildly irritable or show some other personality change; others will develop cognitive problems that range from mild forgetfulness to severe dementia. Depression, mania, and paranoid psychosis have all been reported.

Evaluation

A routine blood test will usually find that the red blood cells are larger than normal, hence one name for this disease, macrocytic anemia. Because other disorders can cause macrocytic anemia, accurate diagnosis must include laboratory measurement of serum cobalamin.

Outcome

PA takes its name from one of the meanings of "pernicious:" deadly. But with adequate treatment, a normal life span can be expected. Because the problem is usually one of malabsorption, oral vitamins are inadequate except in megadoses that are expensive and difficult to manage. But vitamin B_{12} administered by intramuscular injection (monthly, once therapy has been established) reverses most of the symptoms. Some PA patients develop cancer of the stomach, necessitating a lifetime of careful follow-up.

PHEOCHROMOCYTOMA

Occurrence	Age of onset	Gender	Refer to
Uncommon	Young adult to middle age	Slight female excess	Surgeon
What: A usually benign tumor that, under physical stress, secretes catecholamines			
Physical: Attacks of headache, sweating, palpitations, nausea, high blood pressure			
Mental: Anxiety, panic attacks			

Upon being diagnosed as having a tumor, almost anyone would feel anxious. But pheochromocytomas typically cause severe anxiety in people who have no idea they are ill. The reason is that these small, usually benign tumors produce epinephrine and norepinephrine. These two chemicals belong to the group called catecholamines, and their work as neurotransmitters, among other tasks, involves the production of anxiety symptoms and high blood pressure.

Usually located in the abdomen, pheochromocytomas are vulnerable to being jostled by sudden movement (vigorous exercise, or even sneezing). When so disturbed, they inject pulses of catecholamines into the bloodstream, thereby causing symptoms to occur in a paroxysmal or episodic manner. Although these attacks usually occur with some frequency, in some patients weeks or months go by between attacks.

This unusual disease accounts for only about 1 in 1,000 hypertensive patients. Although it can occur at any age, it is most common in young to middle-aged adults. Women develop it slightly more often than do men.

Physical Symptoms

Beginning suddenly and lasting usually for an hour or less, these episodes are characterized by the symptoms of severe high blood pressure: headache, excessive sweating, nausea, vomiting, pallor, and heart palpitations. These patients may complain of a variety of other somatic (body) symptoms that include blurred vision, chest pain, dizziness, faintness, flushing, paresthesias, rapid pulse, shortness of breath, and trouble swallowing. The overall picture can resemble thyrotoxicosis.

Note that although the symptoms usually occur episodically, in more than half the patients, blood pressure is elevated between, as well as during, episodes.

Mental Symptoms

In a few patients, panic attacks or other symptoms of anxiety may be prominent. These symptoms can include profound anxiety, fatigue, weakness, and even the sense of impending doom. The overall resulting picture can mimic many different mental disorders, including panic disorder and other anxiety disorders, as well as somatization disorder. Note that the symptoms of pheochromocytoma are often precipitated by *physical* stress, as compared to symptoms of anxiety disorders that are often caused by *mental* distress.

Evaluation

A 24-hour urine specimen obtained during the time when the patient is having symptoms will reveal high catecholamine levels.

Outcome

Surgical removal of the tumor is curative. Of course, the patient's condition must be correctly diagnosed first. But because pheochromocytoma can so closely mimic other causes of physical and mental symptoms, it often happens that the correct diagnosis is not made until autopsy.

PNEUMONIA

Occurrence	Age of onset	Gender	Refer to
Common	See text	Males predominate	Internist
What: Infection of the lungs			
Physical: Fever, cough, chest pain			
Mental: Delirium, anxiety, panic attacks			

Pneumonia isn't a disease; it's a collection of diseases, infections of the lung caused by any of many different microorganisms. Of course, this definition would also apply to bronchitis, so here is the difference: Think of the lung as a tree that appears to be hanging upside down. Bronchitis is an infection of the trunk and major branches; pneumonia affects the twigs and leaves. When enough twigs and leaves become involved, gas exchange can no longer take place, and the organism dies, hence, pneumonia's wry appellation, "the old man's friend."

The organisms that cause pneumonia are sometimes carried to the lung through the bloodstream from other parts of the body. But more often, the source of the infection is much closer to the lung: globs of infectious material originating in the mouth or throat that are inhaled, often when the person is asleep. The culprit may be a sore throat or dental plaque—people with no teeth are less likely to contract certain types of pneumonia. Such aspiration is more likely when a person's level of consciousness is reduced, as by intoxication, seizures, or strokes. These facts should make you want to drink less, take an aspirin a day, and brush your teeth! Other risk factors include smoking, drug abuse, and other disease such as cancer, diabetes, and positive HIV status.

Although pneumonia can occur in patients of any age, most series indicate a predominance of males. The consequences of pneumonia are far more serious in the elderly patient.

Physical Symptoms

Pneumonia usually presents in one of two ways: typical and nontypical. The more typical picture, especially characteristic of patients with bacterial pneumonia, is a rapid onset of fever, a cough that brings up sputum, shortness of breath (or hyperventilation), and chest pain that is noticeable each time the patient takes a breath.

The nontypical pneumonia begins more gradually and the cough is dry (without sputum production). These patients will often complain of symptoms that seem to originate outside of the chest area: headache, fatigue, sore throat, nausea, vomiting, and diarrhea.

Mental Symptoms

Although mental symptoms don't develop in the vast majority of pneumonia patients, they can occur under certain circumstances. Delirium is a possibility in patients who are gravely ill, especially when pneumonia-causing bacteria invade the bloodstream (bacteremia). Delirium is also more likely to occur in older patients who fail to develop fever or cough with a pneumonia.

Any condition that leads to rapid, shallow respirations will reduce carbon dioxide in the blood. This in turn can cause symptoms of anxiety, even panic attacks. Restlessness and rapid respirations, not usual in most pneumonia patients, may occur in those with immunological deficiency.

Evaluation

As was true nearly a century ago, an X-ray film of the chest will reveal most cases of pneumonia.

Outlook

Most cases of pneumonia are readily treatable with antibiotics and other measures. Mental symptoms, because they indicate the presence of more severe, underlying disease, carry an ominous prognosis.

PORPHYRIA

Occurrence	Age of onset	Gender	Refer to
Uncommon	Rare before puberty	Equal	Hematologist
What: Disorder of porphyrin metabolism			
Physical: Abdominal pain, dark urine, nausea, vomiting, constipation, rapid heartbeat, sweating, tremors, muscle weakness, seizures			
Mental: Depression or euphoria, anxiety, delirium, psychosis			

The King was 50 and gravely ill. He complained of intense abdominal pain, and he became distractible and irritable. As his activity level escalated, he became abusive, even fighting physically with his attendants. He could not sleep. An attendant noted that his urine had a dark, almost blue color, which his doctor dismissed as irrelevant. He became delusional, believing that the capital city had been drowned in a deluge. He was bustled off into royal seclusion and treated for madness, while his son ruled as regent.

The King was George III of England, and his illness was not schizophrenia or manic–depressive disease, but a metabolic disease known as porphyria. Porphyrins are precursors of hemoglobin that are produced at many sites in the body. The livers of patients who inherit a particular autosomal dominant defect sometimes produce vast quantities of porphyrins. When they accumulate in the body, they can produce the symptoms suffered by King George III.

Usually these symptoms require a trigger to set them off. Precipitants include low-calorie diets, surgery, infections, and a variety of drugs that include barbiturates, alcohol, estrogens, antiseizure medications, some antidepressants, and a host of sedatives and other medications.

George was in select company: Only about 1 in 20,000 people has porphyria.

Physical Symptoms

The most characteristic symptom is abdominal pain, which is usually steady and not well localized. Pain is often accompanied by other gastrointestinal symptoms, including nausea, vomiting, abdominal distention, and constipation. When left to stand, the urine turns dark; patients may complain of painful urination and inability to pass urine. Overactivity of the sympathetic nervous system can produce symptoms of rapid heartbeat, tremors, restlessness, excessive sweating, and raised blood pressure. The peripheral nervous system can be damaged, inducing motor weakness that can even include paralysis of the muscles of respiration; some patients also report sensory loss. If seizures develop, they can be extremely difficult to treat, because the usual anticonvulsant medications worsen the underlying disease process.

Mental Symptoms

Anxiety symptoms, depression, and other emotional states (King George seemed almost manic at times) may develop rapidly. When he was 27, George had suffered from an episode of depression, during which he was not psychotic. Like George, some patients have difficulty with insomnia. Disorientation may occur, but the psychotic symptoms of delusions and hallucinations usually develop late.

Porphyria is a great imitator. It has led astray more knowledgeable physicians than those who attended King George back in 1788. A few decades ago, a well-known American psychiatrist wrote an entire book that discussed George's "manic–depressive" illness.

Evaluation

The blood and urine will contain markedly increased concentrations of the product of metabolism called porphobilinogen.

Outlook

Although patients can die if left untreated and respiratory paralysis ensues, most, like George, recover. George ultimately regained his throne, but in his later years, probably unrelated to his earlier disease, he became senile. Once again, his son served as regent, this time for nearly a decade.

POSTOPERATIVE STATES

Occurrence	Age of onset	Gender	Refer to
Frequent	Any age	No data	Psychiatrist
What: Mental illness caused by physiological and/or psychological stress of surgery			
Physical: Depends on site of operation			
Mental: Delirium, psychosis, depression, anxiety			

Picture yourself in this predicament. You wake up in a room you've never seen before. You're too weak to move and too sick to protest. Everyone you meet wears a mask; not a single pair of eyes looks familiar. You have tubes in your mouth and in your nose; you can't eat and you can't speak. Somewhere, everywhere, your body hurts. Your limbs are immobilized, so you can't even scratch when you itch. You hear a beeping sound every time your heart beats; sometimes it beats too fast; sometimes it seems to stop completely. The illumination never changes, so you can't tell whether you've been in this fix for an hour, a day, or a week or more.

In circumstances like these, you might think, anyone would become unbalanced. But in fact, mental complications afflict only a minority of those who have just had major surgery. It is especially likely (up to one-third) in those who have had cardiac surgery, but it may also occur after transplantation surgery or brain operations.

Postoperative delirium (when a mental disorder occurs, it is almost always a delirium) generally appears 2–5 days after surgery, following a relatively lucid interval. The symptoms are most likely to occur in older patients, in those who have had a history of alcohol abuse or a relatively fragile cognitive state preoperatively, and in those with serious physical illness who have had relatively long operations.

Physical Symptoms

Other than general symptoms such as pain, these will vary depending upon the site and nature of the operation.

Mental Symptoms

Although patients are sometimes diagnosed as having depression, anxiety, or psychosis, these symptoms are almost invariably due to a delirium, which can be of either the agitated or somnolent type. By definition, problems focusing or maintaining attention will be found in all such patients. Many will experience the phenomenon of sundowning, in which agitation and misperceptions increase during the nighttime hours. Illusions, frank hallucinations, or full-blown persecutory delusions may occur. Fear and disorientation may make patients try to remove IVs, catheters, or other essential tubing.

Evaluation

Although all body fluids will usually be checked for evidence that fluids or chemicals need either to be eliminated or replenished, or to exclude infection or metabolic disturbance, diagnosis is usually based on history and MSE.

Outlook

Postoperative delirium usually improves quickly and resolves within a few days. Resolution may be hastened by orienting procedures, and by having family or friends sit with the patient.

PREMENSTRUAL SYNDROME

Occurrence	Age of onset	Gender	Refer to
Common	Teens to 30s	Female	Gynecologist
What: Syndrome caused by hormonal changes that occur during menstrual cycle			
Physical: Weight gain, breast pain and tenderness, edema, sleep and appetite change, fatigue			
Mental: Anxiety, depression, irritability, poor concentration			

For what is perhaps the most common syndrome in this book, premenstrual syndrome (PMS) is in a peculiar position. Many patients who think they have it, don't. A lot of patients who do have it don't get diagnosed, because their clinicians don't think about it. And, although the people who write the manuals keep coming up with different names (DSM-III-R: late luteal phase dysphoric disorder; DSM-IV: premenstrual dysphoric disorder) to appease political pressure groups that consider the diagnosis an affront to womankind, most sufferers themselves continue to refer to it as PMS. Finally, no one knows why some women suffer so intensely, whereas others hardly know when they are premenstrual. Older ideas about a hormonal imbalance haven't panned out, but a genetic factor has been postulated.

According to research studies, most women of childbearing age have some PMS-like symptoms with their menstrual cycles. But only about 1 in 20 has symptoms severe enough that they should be treated. Although PMS can begin at any age, the search for diagnosis is most likely to begin when the woman is in her 30s.

Several social factors may prevent women from seeking care for PMS: It has been the butt of jokes; some may fear that they will be seen as weak, especially as compared with men; and PMS has even been used in court as a defense for crimes as serious as murder.

Physical Symptoms

Although the criteria of the various DSMs require only mental symptoms, most clinicians regard physical symptoms as important to the diagnosis. You could fill several pages with the symptoms that have been ascribed to PMS; those that occur with some frequency can be stated much more succinctly. They include pain and tenderness in the breasts. Weight gain of several pounds may be experienced as "bloating" of the abdomen or swelling of the ankles (edema). Sleep and appetite may also change up or down from what is usual for the individual. Some patients experience headache or joint or muscle pain. Contrary to popular supposition, pain with menses (dysmenorrhea) is *not* considered a symptom of PMS. And a number of medical conditions (such as asthma, migraine, and seizure disorders) worsen around the time of menstruation.

Whatever symptoms the patient experiences, it is their regular appearance and disappearance with "the time of the month" that distinguishes PMS. Typically, symptoms begin a week or so before the menses and abate once the menstrual flow actually begins, but individual patterns may vary somewhat. Women who have had a hysterectomy do not have menstrual flow but may ovulate anyway; they are still at risk for PMS symptoms.

Mental Symptoms

Patients most often complain of fatigue; the subjective feelings of anxiety and depression are also frequently reported. Other mood symptoms include irritability or anger, sudden tearfulness, and excessive sensitivity to rejection.

Add the sleep and appetite problems mentioned earlier to decreased energy, trouble concentrating, and loss of interest in usually pleasurable activities, and you will understand why the diagnosis of a primary mood disorder is often erroneously made. Another clinical error to avoid: A patient whose genuine mood or anxiety disorder worsens around the time of menstruation should not be diagnosed as having PMS unless the mood disorder has been successfully treated first. Finally, be careful to avoid accepting the patient's self-diagnosis: As many as half of patients who think they have PMS actually can be diagnosed instead as having a different mental condition, such as a mood disorder.

Other behaviors sometimes associated with PMS are bulimia, psychosis, and even criminal behaviors such as shoplifting.

Evaluation

Although no specific lab tests will confirm the diagnosis, carefully charting weight gain, morning temperature, and symptoms through several cycles may help.

Outcome

For most patients, PMS is more uncomfortable and distracting than it is serious; for some, suicide attempts, accidents, and even criminal behavior may increase during the premenstrual time. Untreated, severe cases tend to worsen with time but abate at menopause.

PRION DISEASE

Occurrence	Age of onset	Gender	Refer to
Rare	Middle age to old age	Equal	Neurologist
What: Disease probably spread by ingestion of infected meat			
Physical: Difficulty walking, tremor, muscle rigidity, hypokinesia			
Mental: Anxiety, poor concentration, dementia			

Okay, so you're unlikely to see a case of kuru, that is, unless your clients happen to include natives of New Guinea who practice ritual cannibalism. Characterized by rapidly progressive dementia and incoordination of gait and other movements, kuru once occurred in about 1% of certain tribal populations in New Guinea. By eating the brains of the dead, these unfortunates also ingested the proteinaceous infectious particles, or prions (pronounced PREE-on), that infected human chromosome number 20, thus transmitting the disease.

With the decline of ritual cannibalism, kuru has almost entirely disappeared, even in New Guinea. But another so-called transmissible neurodegenerative disease, Creutzfeldt–Jakob disease (CJD), continues to be found, though rarely, worldwide.

Although CJD usually begins in middle age or later, in recent years a number of patients in England were found who were much younger—none were older than 42, and some were only teenagers. In the mid-1990s near-hysteria broke out when it was suggested that these cases of CJD were related to bovine spongiform encephalopathy ("mad cow disease"), and that British livestock might be infected with prion disease. Members of Parliament battered one another with accusations, and other nations in the European Common Market boycotted British beef. Eventually, entire herds of cattle were slaughtered and burned, and the fast-food industry in Great Britain took a terrific financial hit. Infectious diseases are an obvious problem for patients and caregivers, but, poorly handled, they also affect the political economies of countries and even entire continents.

Although 10–15% of CJD cases occur in families and are probably inherited as autosomal (not sex-linked) dominants, most occur sporadically. CJD does not appear to be transmitted between human beings by any of the usual body fluid routes, but there have been reported a few cases of transmission through corneal transplant prior to 1988 when it was last used, or therapeutic human growth hormone derived from cadavers. In the mid-1990s, over 1,000 people who had received blood products that *might* have been contaminated with CJD were notified of that fact. As of this writing, I know of no persons who have themselves fallen ill.

Physical Symptoms

Some patients are seen first by a neurologist due to the characteristic difficulty with walking known as cerebellar ataxia. Over 90% eventually develop myoclonus (the sudden contraction of a muscle or group of muscles). The tremor, muscular rigidity, and poverty of motion (hypokinesia) typical of parkinsonism may be encountered in later stages. Other symptoms include headache, dizziness, seizures, and sudden, short-lived blindness.

Mental Symptoms

Early symptoms can include anxiety, fatigue, and poor concentration or slowed thinking. The patient's mood may become quite labile; visual hallucinations may ensue. As the disease progresses, loss of memory and rapidly progressive dementia are almost universal. Most patients have one or more mental symptoms as an initial symptom of the disease.

Evaluation

The single, most valuable laboratory test is the EEG, which in up to 95% of cases will show a characteristic slow-wave background with superimposed sharp waves.

Outlook

There is no treatment other than symptomatic, and death is inevitable, usually within a few months.

PROGRESSIVE SUPRANUCLEAR PALSY

Occurrence	Age of onset	Gender	Refer to
Uncommon	50s or later	About equal	Neurologist
What: Degenerative disorder of central nervous system			
Physical: Double vision, paralysis of gaze, unsteady gait, stiffness			
Mental: Apathy, labile mood, dementia			

Over the years, clinicians have devised a number of ways to say, "I don't know the cause of this condition." It can be *idiopathic* (literally, "individual disease"); it can be *primary* (as in a primary mood disorder). Clinicians who treat children distinguish between disorders that are *developmental* and those that are acquired. Some disorders, such as hypertension, are called *essential,* referring to the notion that their pathology is in the essence of the disease and not due to another illness. An older but perhaps more honest term is *cryptogenic* (literally, "hidden cause").

Any of these expressions would suit progressive supranuclear palsy (PSP), a degenerative disorder of the nervous system, whose cause no one knows. Hidden infections have been sought without success; the disorder does not seem to run in families. Its symptoms are somewhat suggestive of Parkinson's disease, but, affecting only about 1 in 100,000 adults, it is much less common. It usually first appears when patients are middle-aged or older.

Physical Symptoms

An early symptom may be an unsteady gait that comes and goes; later on, the patient may feel unbalanced, unexpectedly falling backward or back-pedaling in an effort to remain upright.

Another early symptom stems from partial paralysis of the muscles that move the eyeball. At first, the patient may complain of double vision; later, there may be an inability to direct the gaze downward. (The cause is not in groups, or nuclei, of cells that control these muscles, located in the brain stem, but in higher brain centers, hence the rather clumsy name of this disorder.)

Later symptoms include an overall slowing of motion and stiffening of muscles. Patients whose gaze is paralyzed often cannot even flex the neck to look downward. What was initially a decreased volume of the voice may become difficulty speaking clearly. Even swallowing can be affected. Some patients also develop sleep apnea. Infrequently, there may be a mild tremor that occurs when the extremities are lying quietly at rest.

Mental Symptoms

Around half of these patients become demented—they think slowly and forget quickly. The dementia may show itself initially as mere apathy. In perhaps a third, pseudobulbar affect develops, a sort of "emotional incontinence" in which the patient may laugh or cry without adequate provocation. When depression or anxiety symptoms occur, they are usually mild. Bipolar disorder and psychosis are rare.

Evaluation

On CT exam of the brain, the pons and midbrain will appear atrophied.

Outlook

Unhappily, there is no known effective treatment for PSP. With progression, some patients completely lose the ability to speak or to direct their gaze. Death usually occurs within 6–10 years.

PROTEIN ENERGY MALNUTRITION

Occurrence	Age of onset	Gender	Refer to
Common	Bimodal (see text)	About equal	Internist
What: Starvation due to the lack of adequate protein in diet			
Physical: Weight loss, low vital signs, lethargy, skin shiny and red, hair dry and thin, peripheral neuropathy			
Mental: Apathy, cognitive change, occasional psychosis			

It's a little hard to imagine malnutrition in a country where nearly half of all adults are overweight. We associate malnutrition with Third World countries, concentration camps, and the Donner–Reed party, who, stranded by California snows in 1849, ultimately dined upon one another.

Of course, malnutrition means more than simply going hungry. It implies the prolonged absence of the variety of dietary substances needed to sustain good health. Well-fed people whose diets lack certain elements (iodine) or vitamins (thiamin, niacin), or who cannot absorb important nutritional factors (vitamin B_{12}) also may be said to be malnourished.

However, this section is concerned with a form of starvation due to the inadequate intake of protein, which cannot be synthesized from either fat or carbohydrate. Though common enough worldwide—perhaps 150 million children suffer from protein energy malnutrition (PEM)—in America and in other Western countries are found only occasional extreme examples of this disorder. These include patients with anorexia nervosa, for whom the relationship is obvious; alcoholics, who may derive nearly all of their calories from a diet that contains no protein whatsoever; and the elderly, whose food intake may be compromised by Alzheimer's disease, apathy, depression, or a variety of physical infirmities that interfere with their ability to obtain, prepare, chew, swallow, or digest their food.

But even in highly advanced Western countries, more subtle evidence of PEM can be found in numerous children who are reared in poverty and relative neglect. Older theories held that

it was brain damage alone that mediated intellectual development in such children. More recent evidence suggests rather that
several interacting factors lead to cognitive deficits:

- The brain's physical structure is delayed or stunted in its
  growth.
- Lower than normal energy levels render the child too
  lethargic to explore the environment.
- Adults may perceive small, malnourished children as
  younger than their chronological age, and hence fail to
  stimulate them for maximal development.
- Poor communities may offer little to stimulate any child,
  well nourished or not.

Physical Symptoms

In adults, the most common symptoms of PEM are loss of weight
and subcutaneous fat. In advanced disease, skin loses its elasticity
and may become shiny and reddened. Some patients develop
peripheral neuropathy (loss of motor or sensory functioning). A
pregnant woman may deliver a baby with low birth weight. Hair
is dry, dull, and thin. Constipation may develop; there is a
general lowering of body vital signs (blood pressure, heart rate,
and temperature).

But children, who are most at risk for this disease, may
develop the even more classical picture of the severe type of
protein deficiency known in Ghana as kwashiorkor, which means
literally "condition encountered in the displaced child." Its
symptoms include bloated belly, wasted limbs, and thinning,
reddish hair. Puberty and general development may be delayed.

Mental Symptoms

PEM patients are typically lethargic, often apathetic, and may
give the appearance of depression. Psychotic symptoms are
occasionally noted. Of course, the chicken-and-egg question must
be sorted out for malnourished adults, many of whom may have
inadequate food intake based on Alzheimer's disease, mood
disorder, or schizophrenia.

Children suffer from a variety of mental and emotional problems: lowered IQ, decreased cognitive ability, and lack of progress in school. They speak and play less well than their adequately nourished peers.

Evaluation

History and physical examination often provide the most useful (and readily obtainable) evidence of PEM. Serum protein levels will help confirm the diagnosis.

Outcome

Restoration of adequate diet alone may not correct the deficits mentioned earlier. Concentration camp survivors have carried symptoms of peripheral neuropathy with them for years; children may never attain expected full growth. Some studies indicate that adequate psychosocial stimulation may be an additional factor needed to ensure that renourished PEM children catch up to peers in intellectual growth and development. And, of course, once the child reaches adulthood, lost height can never be regained.

PULMONARY THROMBOEMBOLISM

Occurrence	Age of onset	Gender	Refer to
Frequent	Older people	Females predominate	Pulmonologist
What: Blood clots formed in the deep veins of the leg travel to the lungs			
Physical: Shortness of breath, faintness, chest pain, coughing up blood			
Mental: Anxiety, delirium			

A thrombus is a blood clot; an embolus is a blood clot that has broken away from the spot where it formed to lodge somewhere else. So this discussion is about blood clots that form (almost always) in the deep veins of a person's legs and end up in the lung. Before they break loose, such clots are called deep vein thromboses, or DVTs, and after they have traveled to the lungs they are called pulmonary thromboembolisms, or PTEs.

The experience of PTE is probably frequent, affecting as many as 500,000 Americans each year. Particularly at risk are people who must be immobile for long times—those who have just had babies, heart attacks, or major operations, for example, and those who are obese or use estrogens. At least in part due to the difficulty of recognizing the symptoms and rapidly beginning therapy, treatment of PTE is not always successful. Most of the deaths occur within an hour or two of the event.

Physical Symptoms

Many, perhaps most, cases of PTE are asymptomatic. Of course, when that is the case, by definition, they do not cause disability or death. Even when the event is serious, often the only symptom is shortness of breath that begins suddenly, without apparent explanation. Chest pain and coughing up blood only occur when lung tissue actually dies—an infrequent event, thanks to the lungs' rich oxygen supply. Patients may note faintness (syncope) or rapid heartbeat; those with previously existing congestive heart failure may worsen with PTE.

Although the site of the initial clot may itself be symptom-free, about half the patients will have typical DVT symptoms: pain, swelling, heat and tenderness of the calves, where the blood clots form.

Mental Symptoms

PTE is likely to produce one significant mental symptom: anxiety associated with shortness of breath and hyperventilation. With fat embolus (as from the marrow from a broken bone), delirium and coma may supervene.

Evaluation

Chest X-rays may show subtle evidence of PTE, but definitive diagnosis is with dye contrast venography, which is not easy, cheap, or comfortable. Routine laboratory studies are valueless.

Outlook

For patients who live long enough to seek medical attention, the prognosis is quite good. However, about 1 in 10 isn't that lucky. As stated, the majority probably don't even realize that they have been at risk.

RHEUMATOID ARTHRITIS

Occurrence	Age of onset	Gender	Refer to
Common	30s and 40s	Females predominate	Rheumatologist
What: Immunological disease affecting connective tissue			
Physical: Fatigue, weakness, anorexia, swollen and painful joints			
Mental: Depression, rare psychosis			

In the world of mental disorders, rheumatoid arthritis (RA) is something of a fraud. Even as recently as a generation ago, it was considered to be one of the classic psychosomatic disorders. Clinicians widely believed that it was caused—at the very least, worsened—by factors in the patient's personality that in some way set the stage for developing the painful, often debilitating symptoms. Popular belief has held that depression and other mental disorders are fundamental symptoms of RA, but that assertion, too, is currently in question.

Another of the seemingly endless immunologically related disorders, RA's actual cause is still unknown. People who contract it are genetically predisposed, but it could be precipitated by an infectious agent such as herpes virus. It more often affects women than men (3:1 ratio) and begins during young adulthood; when it develops for the first time in older people, the sex ratio is less extreme. There is also a juvenile form that attacks teenagers and younger children. Persons of all races and in all countries can be affected—about 1% of the world's population in all.

Physical Symptoms

Although we may be tempted to think of RA as just another type of arthritis, it is really a systemic illness that affects multiple organ systems. The early symptoms begin slowly and are generalized: fatigue, weakness, vague aches and pains, and loss of appetite. After several weeks to months, during which clinicians may be puzzled as to diagnosis, the typical joint swelling and pain begin, and the mystery is solved.

Classically, the first sites affected are the knuckles and the proximal interphalangeal (PIP) joints—the first finger joints beyond the knuckle. The second finger joints—distal interphalangeal joints—are spared, God knows why. The joints are painful and stiff, especially first thing in the morning. They hurt more when they move. With time, they swell; after a number of years, the PIP joints remain permanently swollen. Knuckles may deteriorate so badly that the fingers become deviated away from the thumbs (called ulnar deviation)—toward the elbow. Other joints can also become affected, including wrists, ankles, elbows and knees. When large joints such as the knees are affected, they may even feel warm to the touch.

In addition to painful joints, patients may complain of difficulty breathing, and loss of weight and muscle mass. Some will develop fever. In one-fourth or more, nodules will form at the elbows or in other places in the body. Osteoporosis (decreased bone density, increasing the risk for fractures) is common; ulcerative colitis may develop in some.

Mental Symptoms

A large number—perhaps as many as half—of RA patients become depressed. This mood disorder, once thought to be specifically related to the pathology of underlying condition, is now regarded as a complication understandable in the light of any severe chronic illness. It is easy to comprehend why: Patients worry about becoming a burden on family, being unable to work or pay their bills, unable even to sleep or enjoy sex. Although the occasional patient will develop psychosis, this is pretty rare. In fact, very possibly it has nothing to do with the disease itself, but rather is the result of taking medications such as steroids.

Evaluation

Most patients will have an elevation of blood rheumatoid factor (RF), which is caused by antibodies. However, physical symptoms are so typical that the diagnosis becomes obvious as the disease progresses.

Outlook

Prognosis for RA is quite variable. Some patients quickly worsen and become incapacitated. Most remain active for many years. However, after years or even decades of gradual decline, most will show some evidence of incapacity. On average, life expectancy is shortened by as much as 7 years.

SICKLE-CELL DISEASE

Occurrence	Age of onset	Gender	Refer to
Frequent	Early childhood	Equal	Hematologist
What: Recessive gene causes deformed red blood cells in people of African descent			
Physical: Severe pain episodes, fatigue, enuresis			
Mental: Depression, drug dependence, mental retardation			

Some genetic disorders cause havoc in those who are afflicted, yet are maintained in high numbers in the general population. The presumption is that the gene, or genes, in a "dose" too small to produce the symptoms of disease, must confer on the individual some selective advantage to ensure that the genes are passed on from one generation to the next. Mental health workers have struggled for years, without much success, to find such a competitive advantage for schizophrenia. But for many years, it has been known why the trait for sickle-cell anemia has maintained itself. The answer is malaria.

Sickle-cell anemia is carried by a recessive gene for hemoglobin that is present in about 8% of African Americans. Individuals who are heterozygous for the gene (they have one abnormal and one normal gene) will have blood hemoglobin that resists the infection of falciparum malaria, which is endemic in many parts of Africa. In resisting malaria, the heterozygote individual has a competitive advantage over someone with no copy of the sickle-cell gene, which is why it is perpetuated in the population. But when a person inherits two copies, as occurs in just over 1 in 1,000 African American children, there is hell to pay.

The problem develops from the shape of the red blood cell. Normal red blood cells are described as biconcave discs (they look like Life Savers, without an actual hole). This shape allows ready transfer of oxygen from blood to the cells of the body where it is needed; the biconcave shape is also flexible enough that the red cells do not become stuck in the tiny capillaries they must traverse during their journey as the heart propels them from the lungs to the body and back again. But when sickle cells give up their oxygen, their physical shape becomes distorted into a shape something like a saucer. Viewed edge-on through a microscope, it looks like the blade of a sickle, hence their name. This shape is rigid and promotes blood vessel obstruction; clotting, infarction, and tissue death ensue.

Physical Symptoms

The most evident symptom of this disease is sickle-cell crisis, the painful intermittent blockage of tiny blood vessels. The pain can occur in nearly any part of the body, but it most often affects the abdomen, back, chest, and joints. Several precipitants—infections, hot or cold weather—can set off these episodes with astonishing suddenness. Depending on the individual, crises may occur frequently or at great intervals.

Because sickle cells die within about 15 days, instead of the 120 days for normal red blood cells, these patients are often anemic and complain of chronic fatigue. Many such children wet the bed. By adult life, repeated interference with blood supply can produce symptoms of failure of heart, lung, kidney or liver. In addition, sickle-cell patients are at risk for chronic skin ulceration, infection of the bones (sometimes leading to hip fracture), a host of causes of visual loss and, in men, priapism (acute, painful engorgement of the penis with persistent erection). Sickling in the small arteries of the brain can lead to seizures or recurring strokes.

Mental Symptoms

As is true in any severe, chronic childhood illness, depression and social problems are common in sickle-cell patients. Repeated bouts of severe pain may cause dependence on narcotic drugs or the appearance of drug-seeking behavior.

In addition, about 5% of patients suffer from impaired intellectual development.

Evaluation

Sickle-cell crises can mimic other disorders such as appendicitis, pneumonia, or arthritis, so the disease should be kept in mind whenever treating Black patients. Although a routine blood smear may reveal sickle-cell forms, special provocative tests may be necessary.

Outlook

Although mortality in early life is still high, many patients survive to maturity and beyond; the average age at death is now in the mid-40s. Note that people with sickle-cell trait (only one copy of the gene and no disease) have normal life expectancy, no increase in hospitalization rates, and are only rarely inconvenienced by their genetic status.

SLEEP APNEA

Occurrence	Age of onset	Gender	Refer to
Common	Usually after 40	Males predominate	Pulmonologist
What: Potentially lethal, repeated cessation of breathing when asleep			
Physical: Snoring, morning headache			
Mental: Insomnia, daytime drowsiness, depression, irritability, poor concentration			

Snoring has been a real boon to generations of comedy writers and cartoonists. Images of window-rattling snorts and irritated spouses have tickled funny bones worldwide, perhaps for as long as people have told jokes. But one cause of snoring isn't funny at all—it is associated with depression, dementia, and death.

By definition, sleep apnea patients stop breathing when they are asleep. These little cessations of regular breathing last from 10–60 seconds and can occur dozens of times each night. In the most common type of sleep apnea, the patient has a long history of snoring due to tissues of the mouth and throat that partly block incoming air. During a sleep apnea episode, the blockage becomes complete; the patient's chest heaves in the struggle to inhale. Eventually the blockade gives way, and then an extra loud snort ushers in regular breathing. A few minutes later, the entire process is repeated. During periods of sleep apnea, blood oxygen falls and the level of sleep may be disrupted.

In the less common, central type of sleep apnea, the patient does not snore but simply stops making any effort to breathe. Men with central sleep apnea may complain especially of hypersomnia; women with this type of sleep apnea may complain of insomnia. Why there would be such a difference in the two sexes is beyond me.

Sleep apnea affects anywhere from 1% to 10% of the general population. It is especially likely to occur after the age of 40. Although it is far more common in males (by about 20 to 1), after menopause, the incidence in females increases. Note that most people who snore do *not* have sleep apnea.

Physical Symptoms

The snoring itself never disturbs the snorer, who is asleep. It may constitute a significant problem, however, for bedmates, roommates, housemates, and, if the cartoonists are to be at all believed, neighbors down the street. These patients, many of whom are obese, may also have high blood pressure and irregular or slowed heartbeat. During the night, they may sweat heavily and kick at bedclothes and bed partners. Some also complain of impotence and morning headache. Nocturia (arising at night to urinate) is often present; enuresis (bedwetting) is an occasional symptom.

Mental Symptoms

Interrupted sleep leads to complaints of daytime sleepiness and cognitive impairment that includes distractibility, and problems with memory, perception, or orientation. Patients who are both obese and sleepy during the day are sometimes said to have Pickwickian syndrome, named for the somnolent fat boy in Dickens's *The Pickwick Papers*. Some patients experience hallucinations when going to sleep. The apneic periods may be associated with severe anxiety, ongoing depression, or irritability.

Evaluation

Sleep polysomnography can confirm this diagnosis, though a bed partner's report of the typical snoring–not snoring pattern is nearly diagnostic.

Outcome

Treatment with continuous positive airway pressure (CPAP) through a mask can improve the lot of many of these patients and may even save the lives of some.

SYPHILIS

Occurrence	Age of onset	Gender	Refer to
Uncommon	See text	Males predominate	Internist
What: Sexually transmitted infection			
Physical: Chancre (genital ulcer, primary stage), rash (secondary), multiple neurological problems (tertiary)			
Mental: Fatigue, personality change, mood disorder, psychosis, dementia			

One morning, following a night of far too much champagne, young Randolph Churchill, the future father of Winston Churchill, awakened by the side of a snaggletoothed crone. Without the slightest memory of how he had gotten there (or what had transpired), he fled in terror. Despite a disinfectant prescribed by his physician, 3 weeks later he developed a genital ulcer known as chancre, the first stage of syphilis. Years later, he entered Parliament and quickly rose to become Chancellor of the Exchequer. But until he died at the age of 45, Lord Randolph Churchill's life was defined by the torment and humiliation of a disease that may have deprived Great Britain of a Prime Minister.

Ten years into his illness, he suffered from fevers and recurrent headaches. His personality changed, becoming irritable and irascible. He might hardly speak to old friends from whom he had been nearly inseparable a short time before. These symptoms waxed and waned as he became increasingly erratic and moody. His speeches in the House of Commons became incomprehensible. Paranoia ensued; he threatened his wife with a loaded revolver. At one port of call on a world cruise arranged to get him away from London, he went berserk and bought the entire contents of a shop. He finally returned home a month before his death, demented and groaning with pain.

The cause of all this misery is a tiny spirochete called *Treponema pallidum,* a one-celled microbe that thrives on moist tissues. It is transmitted directly from one person to another through sexual contact. Penicillin has greatly reduced the number of persons who go on to develop the tertiary disease, at various times called general paresis of the insane, dementia paralytica, and central nervous system lues. Even so, it affects around 3 per 100,000 population each year.

Physical Symptoms

The initial symptom, the ulcerous chancre, is followed within a couple of months by headache, fever, fatigue, sore throat, a generalized skin rash (raised, blotchy, red rash, particularly noteworthy in that it even extends to the palms and soles), and swollen lymph nodes. After a few weeks of these symptoms, then nothing further for perhaps a dozen years or more, in around one-third of people who have not been adequately treated with antibiotics, the symptoms of neurosyphilis begin. These include the following forms:

- *Meningeal syphilis.* Arising as early as a year after infection, it produces headache, stiff neck, nausea, vomiting, and seizures.
- *Meningovascular syphilis.* After 1–10 years, headache, dizziness, insomnia precede symptoms of stroke. This form is not common.
- *General paresis.* After 20 years, reflexes become hyperactive, and the pupil of the eye loses its ability to react when a light is shone upon it. Tremors may develop in the face and tongue; the patient may have difficulty writing or even speaking clearly.
- *Tabes dorsalis.* Twenty-five years or more down the road, loss of myelin (therefore, loss of functioning) of parts of the spinal cord causes trouble. The patient develops a wide-based gait with characteristic slapping of the feet as they are brought down with each step. There may occur loss of reflexes and bladder control, impotence, lightning pains and loss of other senses in the legs, including those of temperature, position, and deep pain. The joints may become so loose that the knee can be moved in directions normally impossible (called Charcot's joint).

Half or more of patients with long-untreated syphilis develop disease of the heart and great blood vessels. Peak incidence of primary syphilis (chancre) is in the 15- to 34-year-olds. The age of onset of neurosyphilis will be during early to mid-adult life.

Mental Symptoms

For generations, because of its ability to mimic most any mental syndrome, neurosyphilis has been called the great imitator. Early symptoms include fatigue, forgetfulness, irritability, personality change, and tremor. Anyone like Randolph Churchill, unfortunate enough to remain untreated, may suffer from deteriorating judgment, loss of insight, delusions, or hallucinations. Manic

grandiosity, once regarded as the classical symptom of this scourge, is now rare.

There is also a juvenile form of neurosyphilis, transmitted from mother to fetus during gestation. These children can suffer from cognitive impairment, delayed development, and regressed behavior.

Evaluation

Diagnosis is by serum screening test (once it was the Wasserman test, now it is the venereal disease research laboratory [VDRL] test), followed by the more definitive FTA-ABS (serum fluorescent treponeme antibody absorption) test. Even after treatment, some patients will remain seropositive, perhaps for a lifetime.

Outlook

Trading sexual favors for crack cocaine has caused an increase in untreated, primary-stage syphilis (as well as other sexually transmitted diseases) in certain populations, notably young Black men who live in inner cities. Untreated, perhaps 10% of those who become infected will develop neurosyphilis.

Thanks to penicillin, neurosyphilis is now an unusual diagnosis. Untreated, the tiny microbe that killed Randolph Churchill, Scott Joplin, and Franz Schubert will relentlessly pursue its unfortunate host through seizures, dementia, mutism, and death. Even when given after the mental symptoms of neurosyphilis have begun, the patient can expect improvement in the ability to think and perform the activities of daily living.

SYSTEMIC INFECTION

Occurrence	Age of onset	Gender	Refer to
Common	Any age	Males predominate	Internist

What: The brain is affected by infections occurring outside the head

Physical: Fever, nausea, vomiting, diarrhea, abdominal pain, cough, painful breathing, jaundice, rash, itching, genital discharge, pain

Mental: Delirium, anxiety, mild depression

Infections that occur in the head, where they can directly affect the brain, are extremely serious. (They are covered in other sections in this volume.) Fortunately, they are relatively uncommon. On the other hand, infections that originate elsewhere in the body are so common that everyone has them from time to time. Fortunately, these do not usually produce mental symptoms; those that do are often found in patients with especially vulnerable brains—those of the very young and of the very old. IV-drug users are especially susceptible to systemic bacterial and viral infections; travelers abroad are especially vulnerable to infection by intestinal parasites.

Physical Symptoms

Of course, the number and variety of symptoms will depend largely upon the infectious agent and the body part it attacks. I have tried here only to list those symptoms that are relatively more common.

Generalized

These symptoms are not related exclusively to any one organ system. Fever may begin acutely or gradually, depending upon the infectious agent. Fever occurs with many infections but especially with septicemia, when bacteria proliferate in the bloodstream. The fever, which may cause hard, shaking chills (as at the onset of typhus), also commonly speeds up other physiological processes such as heartbeat and respirations. In some diseases, such as tuberculosis, fever may be conspicuously absent. When fever leads to dehydration, thirst ensues.

Gastrointestinal

Nausea and vomiting occur frequently in infections of the upper digestive tract. Intestinal parasites and some bacteria often cause diarrhea; it is likely to be watery (shigella, cholera), but diarrhea may sometimes be bloody. When a patient cannot replace body fluids fast enough, prolonged diarrhea yields dehydration that in turn produces weakness and lethargy. The increased intestinal

motility associated with the diarrhea may produce abdominal pain, which can also occur with abscess of the peritoneum (the lining of the intestines and abdomen). Blood pressure may fall, especially with a septicemia due to the meningococcus, a common cause of meningitis. Mononucleosis produces sore throat. Infected rectum or anus can produce a painful straining at stool, called tenesmus.

Cardiopulmonary

Patients with infected lungs usually cough. The cough may be dry or produce sputum (tuberculosis). Impaired gas exchange can produce rapid respirations, and the mere act of breathing can be painful (called pleuritic pain).

Skin

When an infection such as pneumonia impedes air exchange in the lungs, the skin may look purplish (cyanosis). If the liver is involved, as in hepatitis, the waste products it normally excretes accumulate in other organs, including the skin. Then, the skin takes on a yellow hue, called jaundice. Other color changes may include generalized reddening of the skin, purple blotches that can occur with sepsis, and a variety of rashes that range from the blotches of measles down to the pencil-point petechiae of Rocky Mountain spotted fever. Skin manifestations of dehydration include decreased sweating and loss of tissue turgor (or stiffness—think of wilted lettuce). Some skin lesions (genital herpes) cause itching.

Genitourinary

GU infections may be signaled by a discharge of pus from the penis or the vagina (e.g., gonorrhea). Then, the mere act of urinating can be excruciating. A woman may experience abdominal pain due to infected ovaries or Fallopian tubes; a man may complain of painful testicles. Although pain with intercourse can be due to a vaginal infection, the cause is usually something different.

Mental Symptoms

Although a few days of low mood is common enough with infectious diseases (remember how you felt the last time you had the flu), depressive symptoms severe enough for a diagnosis of a major depressive episode are unusual. Patients who have trouble breathing will probably experience anxiety or even panic symptoms; apprehension progressing to agitation has been reported with typhus. But delirium is relatively common, especially with systemic infections that induce septicemia or high fever. Then, disorientation and even hallucinations may become prominent; they may even be the symptoms that cause the patient to seek help. The elderly can experience pneumonia with virtually no physical symptoms at all, only mental symptoms such as delirium.

Recently, tics and obsessive–compulsive symptoms have been found in children who have autoimmune disorders associated with streptococcal infections. The condition has been labeled pediatric autoimmune neuropsychiatric disorders associated with streptococcal infections, or PANDAS.

Evaluation

Depending upon site of infection, physical examination, X-ray, white-blood-cell count, and growing the offending organism on culture medium may be appropriate.

Outcome

As you might imagine, there will be marked variability depending upon the virulence of the pathogen, how soon it was detected, availability of appropriate antibiotic treatment, age of the patient, and the presence of other illnesses. If not appropriately treated, septicemia is often fatal. Fortunately, the vast majority of systemic infections are self-limited, responding well to such measures as aspirin and a day or two away from work.

SYSTEMIC LUPUS ERYTHEMATOSUS

Occurrence	Age of onset	Gender	Refer to
Frequent	Childbearing age	Females predominate	See text
What: Antibodies against the body's own cells cause widespread symptoms			
Physical: Muscle and joint pain, "butterfly" rash, fatigue, fever, anorexia, weight loss, nausea, diarrhea, cough, painful breathing, weakness, pallor			
Mental: Severe depression, delirium, dementia, psychosis			

Systemic lupus erythematosus (SLE) is hardly rare—it may affect as many as 50 out of every 100,000 Americans—but neither is it exactly a household term. It does belong to the family of such well-known diseases as rheumatoid arthritis, myasthenia gravis, and, perhaps, multiple sclerosis. These disorders are called autoimmune, because they appear to come about when the body forms antibodies against components of its own cells. Among these illnesses, SLE is remarkable for the extent of damage and variety of symptoms it can cause.

Because it principally affects women of childbearing age (it is around three times as common as in older women), hormones are thought to play a part in its development. But it also runs in families, and a genetic linkage has been demonstrated. Blacks and Asians are more likely to be affected than Caucasians. Finally, some authors have implicated various environmental precipitants, including sunlight, hair dye, and alfalfa sprouts! Truly, SLE is a disorder to be reckoned with.

Physical Symptoms

If there is a defining experience for SLE patients, it is pain—nearly all have muscle or joint pain. Affected most are wrists, knees, and fingers (less so the terminal joints of the fingers). But the most visible and characteristic manifestation of this disease is the rash that in about half the patients develops across the bridge of the nose and over the cheeks in a characteristic "butterfly" pattern. This rash worsens when exposed to light (photosensitivity).

Patients may complain of feeling fatigued. They may develop fever and lose appetite and weight. Some have nausea and diarrhea. Prey to chest infection, they may develop shortness of breath, a cough, and pain upon breathing. Anemia is a common experience that can show itself as weakness or pallor.

Of the many complications associated with SLE, miscarriage is the most common, affecting one-third or more of pregnancies. Kidney failure, liver failure, or stroke can be the fate of other patients. Around 20% have seizures.

Mental Symptoms

Most SLE patients are affected mentally at one time or another. The trouble is, no one has been sure whether mental disorder has been caused by the disease itself or by medications such as steroids used to treat it. (At least one recent study suggests the former.) In any event, up to half the patients may have symptoms of severe depression, and many have some symptoms of cognitive disorder. It may be a delirium that is associated with the physical complications of the disease, but it is far more likely to be a relatively subtle problem with memory or language. A few patients actually become demented. Psychosis isn't exactly rare; when it occurs, is it due to the disease or its treatment with steroids?

Evaluation

Although not specific for SLE, antinuclear antibodies (ANA) in the blood will characteristically be elevated.

Outcome

Because SLE patients so often have renal disease, the nephrologist is the logical caregiver for many. Older patients with predominately arthritic symptoms should see a rheumatologist. Some teenage patients develop lupus cerebritis and should be referred to a neurologist.

About 25% of patients have such mild disease that they have little or no disability. Overall, around two-thirds survive more than 10 years, but it is hard to predict at the outset who these will be. Disability is common, and there is some evidence that having mental symptoms may worsen the prognosis.

THIAMINE DEFICIENCY

Occurrence	Age of onset	Gender	Refer to
Frequent	Older	Males predominate	Neurologist

What: Inadequate levels of vitamin B1 inhibit many enzymatic reactions			
Physical: Shortness of breath, rapid heartbeat, edema, motor weakness, sensory changes in extremities, nystagmus, paralysis of gaze, trouble walking, fever, vomiting			
Mental: Anxiety, delirium, amnesia			

With improved nutritional information and vitamin supplementation of basic foodstuffs, the great vitamin deficiency scourges, such as scurvy and pellagra, are little more than a memory in developed countries. But the deficiency of thiamine (vitamin B$_1$) remains with us today, though in reduced numbers.

The outer coatings of cereal grains are especially rich in thiamine. That's why whole wheat bread is a better source than white (unless the white flour is enriched), and why deficiency states sometimes occur in people from developing countries who eat milled (white) rice. Because alcohol is especially poor in thiamine, severe neurological syndromes develop in patients who drink so much that they obtain nearly all of their calories from alcohol.

Although in Western societies we believe that we seldom encounter vitamin deficiency, some evidence suggests that it occurs rather frequently, especially among older people. With alcoholism a principal cause of thiamine deficiency in this country, men are at greater risk than are women. Whites are more susceptible than are non-Whites.

Physical Symptoms

Patients with thiamine deficiency may have cardiac or neurological symptoms; most patients will have some of each.

The symptoms of heart disease include shortness of breath upon relatively slight exercise (physicians call this dyspnea on exertion), rapid heartbeat, and swelling of the extremities (dependent edema). Other symptoms of thiamine deficiency include weakness, nausea, and muscle aches and pains.

The disease of the nervous system ("dry beriberi") comes in several parts, usually referred to as peripheral neuropathy, Wernicke's syndrome, and Korsakoff's syndrome. The third I will discuss under Mental Symptoms.

About 80% of the patients develop a "symmetrical peripheral neuropathy of the distal limbs." This translates to motor weakness and sensory changes (numbness, pins-and-needles sensations) of the hands, feet, forearms or lower legs, changes that are about equal on both sides of the body.

Patients with Wernicke's syndrome (also known as Wernicke's encephalopathy) may have generalized symptoms of fever and vomiting, but their neurological symptoms are quite specific. There is nystagmus (a rapid oscillation of the eyeball back and forth), which may be obscured by the fact that, almost always, the muscles that turn the eyeballs in their sockets are partly paralyzed. The result: Gazing to the side can only be accomplished by turning the entire head. Gait is also affected, sometimes to the point that a patient is not able to walk at all without help.

Mental Symptoms

Infrequently, with shortness of breath due to fulminant beriberi heart disease, the patient may become acutely anxious and restless. A much more likely (though still distinctly uncommon) set of symptoms is the delirium that accompanies an acute Wernicke's syndrome. Such patients are inattentive, disoriented, lethargic, and apathetic—they speak little and suffer impaired memory.

As the delirium and acute physical symptoms of Wernicke's syndrome clear, in some patients they will gradually give way to the distinctive memory loss that characterizes Korsakoff's syndrome. Although there may be some loss of memory for past events, what is most impressive is the anterograde amnesia—the inability to form new, permanent memories. Although these patients can recount something that has occurred only seconds earlier, they cannot retain it longer than a few minutes.

Here is a description of this classic, profound amnesia: Someone enters the room, speaks with the patient, and leaves, only to return a few minutes later. But the patient, who doesn't remember that a meeting and conversation has just occurred, is willing to have the entire conversation again! Korsakoff patients are disoriented for time and place and cannot understand their situation (e.g., they may misidentify a hospital room as a library). Sometimes, relatively early in the course of this illness, they may confabulate: They make up facts or stories that attempt to disguise the difficulties they have with memory. However, Korsakoff patients do not have to any considerable extent the apraxia, agnosia, aphasia, or troubles with executive functioning that are required for a diagnosis of dementia (DSM-IV calls this condition an amnestic disorder).

Evaluation

The reliable, modern techniques for identifying CNS pathology, CT scan and MRI, may be completely normal in Wernicke–Korsakoff disease. In any case, the results of examination may come too late if treatment is delayed for a definitive diagnosis. That is why thiamine must be started immediately, by injection, upon the slightest suspicion of deficiency. Thus, patients with alcoholism are routinely treated with large doses of the vitamin, whether or not they truly need it.

Outlook

When the heart disease is severe and acute, the patient will become acutely short of breath, restless, and anxious. Although recovery with vitamin replacement therapy is nothing short of miraculous, death from hemorrhage in the brain comes within hours if treatment is delayed. Nearly one-fifth of hospitalized patients do die of their disease, and many survivors never recover the ability to walk without shuffling.

Although it used to be said that Korsakoff patients never recovered, in fact, about half do. For the remainder, confabulation gradually diminishes, leaving behind the shell of a person for whom all connections between the distant past and a tiny sliver of the present must be forever lost.

WILSON'S DISEASE

Occurrence	Age of onset	Gender	Refer to
Uncommon	Teens–young adulthood	Equal	Neurologist
What: Inherited inability of liver to excrete copper yields toxic buildup			
Physical: Trouble speaking, tremor, spasticity, rigidity, drooling, difficulty swallowing, dystonia			
Mental: Personality change (irritability, disinhibited), depression, psychosis, cognitive disorders			

You probably don't think much about copper as it relates to health, unless you're one of those who tries to ward off arthritis by wearing bracelets made of the stuff. But in Wilson's disease (also known as hepatolenticular degeneration), the body has difficulty excreting copper. Caused by an inborn metabolic error, copper builds up in the liver, the brain, and the eye, creating havoc for the small minority of people who inherit this autosomal recessive gene. It is a disease mainly of young people—the average age of onset is late teens, though first symptoms can appear as late as the 40s. All ethnic groups and races are affected; consanguinity (close blood relationship) is often reported in the parents of these patients. About 1 in 30,000 individuals is affected.

Physical Symptoms

As the site of the principal metabolic defect, liver damage, in the form of either cirrhosis or acute or chronic hepatitis, may lead to liver failure (q.v.) and the need for transplantation. But most of the symptoms are motor, and early symptoms, when not mental, are neurological.

Difficulty speaking (dysarthria) may be an early symptom. Patients may also present with a tremor of the hands or arms. This tremor may occur when the patient is at rest, with a parkinsonian, back-and-forth motion of the fingers and thumb. It can instead be an intention tremor—one that occurs when the patient is trying to do something with the hands, such as touching an object. With elbows bent, some patients may wave their arms up and down in a motion that resembles the beating wings of a bird. Other common motor symptoms include spasticity, rigidity, drooling, difficulty swallowing, and dystonia. Dystonia, which means "abnormal muscle tension," can take the form of a twisting motion of the neck or pelvis. Often, the patient's mouth remains open in a fixed, mirthless smile. Some patients have seizures.

In most patients, copper is eventually deposited in the cornea of the eye. It appears as a golden, speckled ring that may be visible with a hand lens or even the naked eye.

Mental Symptoms

It is still not certain whether the mental symptoms of Wilson's disease are specifically caused by the accumulating copper in the brain or whether they are merely the reaction of a young person to having serious, debilitating symptoms. The former explanation is suggested by the fact that in up to two-thirds of patients, mental symptoms appear before any physical or neurological symptoms.

Personality change has been reported; it is often of the irritable, easy-to-anger type, but some patients become preoccupied with sex and lose their normal social inhibitions. Mood disorders (especially depression) have often been noted, sometimes with suicidal ideas or attempts. Occasionally psychosis, even resembling schizophrenia, may be found; catatonia has been reported. Also noted have been cognitive disorders as severe as dementia, which may be reversible with adequate treatment.

Evaluation

Abnormal liver function tests (liver enzymes, serum bilirubin) are typical. CT scan and MRI may show dilated ventricles in the brain.

Outlook

Early diagnosis, treatment with medication, and adherence to a low-copper diet can improve quality of life and reduce symptom severity. Even symptoms of a cognitive disorder may recede with long-term treatment. Some patients live many years with minimal symptoms and disability.

Part III

SYMPTOM SUMMARIES

This section charts the symptoms I have described in the foregoing text pages. Of course, some symptoms occur much more often than others. In these tables, I have not attempted to indicate frequency, which, after all, is an important feature of groups of patients but less important when considering only one patient at a time. I have tried to include *all* symptoms mentioned in the text, not just those important enough to be included in the brief summary that begins the discussion of each diagnosis in Part II.

It is also important to note that patients may experience many other symptoms than are listed here, or in the text, for that matter. What I have tried to do here is list those that are most common or most important. But always remember that when it comes to healthcare, almost anything is possible.

Symptom definitions are not always as precise as we would like them to be. Often, authors use different terms to mean the same thing, and, in some cases, the same term has various meanings. When the latter is the case, I have tried to make my meaning clear by the use of synonyms. In these tables, I have usually used only one term to stand for several. For example, tiredness and fatigue are used synonymously; inattention stands for poor concentration; restlessness denotes agitation; and so on.

Some terms may seem placed on the wrong page. For example, edema is usually a cardiovascular symptom, but it is also found in hypothyroidism. Is agitation a generalized symptom, or should it be placed with other mental (or, for that matter, neurological) symptoms? Is lethargy a physical symptom, or is it as much attitudinal? Muscle stiffness not only seems more subjective than muscle rigidity, but also the latter implies that agonists and antagonistic muscle groups (e.g., biceps and triceps in the arm) are working at the same time, against one another. These decisions are a matter of taste. I suspect there is something here to offend just about everyone.

Summary of Symptoms: General and Visual

	General symptoms													Eye/vision						
	Weakness	Agitation	Fatigue	Lethargy	Temperature	Obesity	Pain	Blood pressure	Thirst	Feels cold	Feels warm	Breath odor	Sore throat	Blurred	Impaired/blind	Nystagmus	Dilated pupil	Eye signs*	Double vision	Paralyzed gaze
Adrenal insufficiency	×	×						↓												
AIDS	×		×										×		×					
Altitude sickness	×		×	×	↑															
Amyotrophic lateral sclerosis																				
Antidiuretic excess	×	×		×	↑															
Brain abscess				×										×						×
Brain tumor	×			×										×	×	×				
Cancer	×						×									×			×	
Carcinoid syndrome								↓												
Cardiac arrhythmia		×	×					↓												
Cerebrovascular accident		×	×					↑												
Chronic obstructive lung disease			×																	
Congestive heart failure			×							×										
Cryptococcosis	×				↑															
Cushing's syndrome	×	×	×					↑						×						
Deafness																				
Diabetes mellitus									×					×	×				×	
Epilepsy																				
Fibromyalgia			×																	
Head trauma			×	×																
Herpes encephalitis					↑															
Homocystinuria															×					
Huntington's disease																				
Hyperparathyroidism	×	×	×						×											
Hypertensive encephalopathy	×	×	×					↑						×	×					
Hyperthyroidism	×	×	×								×			×				×		

Hypoparathyroidism

Hypothyroidism

Kidney failure

Klinefelter's syndrome

Liver failure

Lyme disease

Ménière's syndrome

Menopause

Migraine

Mitral valve prolapse

Multiple sclerosis

Myasthenia gravis

Neurocutaneous disease

Normal pressure hydrocephalus

Parkinson's disease

Pellagra

Pernicious anemia

Pheochromocytoma

Pneumonia

Porphyria

Postoperative states

Premenstrual syndrome

Prion disease

Progressive supranuclear palsy

Protein energy malnutrition

Pulmonary thromboembolism

Rheumatoid arthritis

Sickle-cell disease

Sleep apnea

Syphilis

Systemic infection

Systemic lupus erythematosus

Thiamine deficiency

Wilson's disease

*Exophthalmos, lid lag, staring, decreased rate of blinking.

193

Summary of Symptoms: Chest and Gastrointestinal

	Chest										Gastrointestinal										
	Shortness of breath	Wheezing	Palpitation	Heart rate	Pain	Cough	Edema	Hyperventilation	Orthopnea	Paroxysmal nocturnal dyspnea	Nausea	Vomiting	Diarrhea	Stool color	Constipation	Appetite	Weight	Bloating	Abdominal pain	Crave salt	Tongue red
Adrenal insufficiency	×										×	×								×	
AIDS	×										×	×	×			→	→		×		
Altitude sickness	×					×										→	→				
Amyotrophic lateral sclerosis	×																				
Antidiuretic excess											×	×				→	→				
Brain abscess											×	×									
Brain tumor												×				→					
Cancer	×															→	→				
Carcinoid syndrome		×											×	Dark		→			×		
Cardiac arrhythmia			×																		
Cerebrovascular accident																					
Chronic obstructive lung disease	×	×				×										→					
Congestive heart failure	×	×					×		×	×	×					→	→				
Cryptococcosis																→	→				
Cushing's syndrome																					
Deafness																					
Diabetes mellitus				←																	
Epilepsy																					
Fibromyalgia																					
Head trauma																					
Herpes encephalitis												×			×						
Homocystinuria																					
Huntington's disease																←					
Hyperparathyroidism											×	×			×	→		×			
Hypertensive encephalopathy			×								×	×							×		
Hyperthyroidism	×		×	←									×			←	→				

Hypoparathyroidism

Hypothyroidism

Kidney failure

Klinefelter's syndrome

Liver failure

Lyme disease

Ménière's syndrome

Menopause

Migraine

Mitral valve prolapse

Multiple sclerosis

Myasthenia gravis

Neurocutaneous disease

Normal pressure hydrocephalus

Parkinson's disease

Pellagra

Pernicious anemia

Pheochromocytoma

Pneumonia

Porphyria

Postoperative states

Premenstrual syndrome

Prion disease

Progressive supranuclear palsy

Protein energy malnutrition

Pulmonary thromboembolism

Rheumatoid arthritis

Sickle-cell disease

Sleep apnea

Syphilis

Systemic infection

Systemic lupus erythematosus

Thiamine deficiency

Wilson's disease

Summary of Symptoms: Genitourinary and Sexual

	Genitourinary											Sexual				
	Increased urination	Urine retention	Small testes	Dark urine	Nocturia	Enuresis	Painful urination	Menses	Breast size	Breast pain, tenderness	Hot flash	Impotence	Low interest	Infertile	Painful intercourse	Priapism
Adrenal insufficiency																
AIDS																
Altitude sickness																
Amyotrophic lateral sclerosis																
Antidiuretic excess																
Brain abscess																
Brain tumor													×			
Cancer													×			
Carcinoid syndrome																
Cardiac arrythmia																
Cerebrovascular accident																
Chronic obstructive lung disease												×	×			
Congestive heart failure												×	×			
Cryptococcosis																
Cushing's syndrome								→				×				
Deafness																
Diabetes mellitus	×															
Epilepsy												×	×			
Fibromyalgia													×			
Head trauma													×			
Herpes encephalitis		×										×				
Homocystinuria																
Huntington's disease																
Hyperparathyroidism																
Hypertensive encephalopathy								→								
Hyperthyroidism												×				

196

Disease	Indicators
Hypoparathyroidism	
Hypothyroidism	× ←
Kidney failure	× × →
Klinefelter's syndrome	× × ←
Liver failure	→ ←
Lyme disease	
Ménière's syndrome	×
Menopause	× × →
Migraine	
Mitral valve prolapse	
Multiple sclerosis	×
Myasthenia gravis	
Neurocutaneous disease	
Normal pressure hydrocephalus	
Parkinson's disease	
Pellagra	
Pernicious anemia	
Pheochromocytoma	
Pneumonia	
Porphyria	× × ×
Postoperative states	×
Premenstrual syndrome	×
Prion disease	
Progressive supranuclear palsy	
Protein energy malnutrition	
Pulmonary thromboembolism	
Rheumatoid arthritis	×
Sickle-cell disease	× × ×
Sleep apnea	× ×
Syphilis	×
Systemic infection	× ×
Systemic lupus erythematosus	×
Thiamine deficiency	
Wilson's disease	

Summary of Symptoms: Skin

	Dark	Pallor	Itching	Hair	Body hair	Lymph nodes	Cyanosis	Jaundice	Reddening	Oily	Acne	Dry	Goiter	Sweating	Warm	Bleeds	Bruising	Ulceration	Rash	See note*
Adrenal insufficiency	×				→															
AIDS																×	×			
Altitude sickness																				
Amyotrophic lateral sclerosis																				
Antidiuretic excess																				
Brain abscess																				
Brain tumor																				
Cancer																				
Carcinoid syndrome																				
Cardiac arrythmia																				
Cerebrovascular accident																				
Chronic obstructive lung disease							×													
Congestive heart failure							×	×												
Cryptococcosis																				
Cushing's syndrome					←				×	×	×									
Deafness																				
Diabetes mellitus														←						
Epilepsy																				
Fibromyalgia																				
Head trauma																				
Herpes encephalitis																				
Homocystinuria				Thin					×											
Huntington's disease																				
Hyperparathyroidism																				
Hypertensive encephalopathy														←						
Hyperthyroidism	×			Fine									×		×					

Hypoparathyroidism

Hypothyroidism

Kidney failure

Klinefelter's syndrome

Liver failure

Lyme disease

Ménière's syndrome

Menopause

Migraine

Mitral valve prolapse

Multiple sclerosis

Myasthenia gravis

Neurocutaneous disease

Normal pressure hydrocephalus

Parkinson's disease

Pellagra

Pernicious anemia

Pheochromocytoma

Pneumonia

Porphyria

Postoperative states

Premenstrual syndrome

Prion disease

Progressive supranuclear palsy

Protein energy malnutrition

Pulmonary thromboembolism

Rheumatoid arthritis

Sickle-cell disease

Sleep apnea

Syphilis

Systemic infection

Systemic lupus erythematosus

Thiamine deficiency

Wilson's disease

*Pedunculated tumor, café au lait spot, sebaceous adenoma, port-wine stain.

199

Summary of Symptoms: Musculoskeletal

	Fractures	Bone pain	Joint pain	Joint swelling	Tall stature	Muscle pain	Muscle rigidity	Muscle stiffness	Muscle tenderness	Muscle wasting	Masked facies
Adrenal insufficiency											
AIDS						X					
Altitude sickness										X	
Amyotrophic lateral sclerosis						X				X	
Antidiuretic excess											
Brain abscess											
Brain tumor											
Cancer											
Carcinoid syndrome											
Cardiac arrythmia											
Cerebrovascular accident											
Chronic obstructive lung disease											
Congestive heart failure											
Cryptococcosis											
Cushing's syndrome											
Deafness										X	
Diabetes mellitus											
Epilepsy											
Fibromyalgia						X		X			
Head trauma									X		
Herpes encephalitis											
Homocystinuria											
Huntington's disease											
Hyperparathyroidism						X				X	
Hypertensive encephalopathy											
Hyperthyroidism										X	

Condition	1	2	3	4	5	6	7	8	9	10
Hypoparathyroidism										
Hypothyroidism		×								
Kidney failure	×					×				
Klinefelter's syndrome					×					
Liver failure			×			×				
Lyme disease			×	×						
Ménière's syndrome										
Menopause	×									
Migraine			×							
Mitral valve prolapse										
Multiple sclerosis										
Myasthenia gravis										
Neurocutaneous disease										
Normal pressure hydrocephalus										
Parkinson's disease							×			×
Pellagra										
Pernicious anemia										
Pheochromocytoma										
Pneumonia										
Porphyria										
Postoperative states										
Premenstrual syndrome			×			×	×			
Prion disease							×			
Progressive supranuclear palsy								×	×	
Protein energy malnutrition										
Pulmonary thromboembolism									×	
Rheumatoid arthritis	×		×			×			×	
Sickle-cell disease	×		×							
Sleep apnea						×				
Syphilis										
Systemic infection										
Systemic lupus erythematosus			×			×				
Thiamine deficiency						×	×			
Wilson's disease							×			

201

Summary of Symptoms: Neurological I

	Fainting/unconsciousness	Abnormal gait	Tremor	Fasciculations	Involuntary movements	Akinesia	Seizures	Swallowing impaired	Speech trouble	Incoordination	Stiff neck	Paralysis	Mutism	Incontinence	Loss of smell	Clumsiness	Focal symptoms	Coma/stupor	Restless legs	Spasticity
Adrenal insufficiency	x																			
AIDS		x					x							x						
Altitude sickness		x		x			x			x										
Amyotrophic lateral sclerosis		x	x	x																
Antidiuretic excess			x				x	x	x											
Brain abscess		x	x				x		x		x	x					x	x		
Brain tumor		x	x				x		x			x		x			x	x		
Cancer																	x			
Carcinoid syndrome																				
Cardiac arrythmia	x																			
Cerebrovascular accident												x	x	x						x
Congestive heart failure																				
Chronic obstructive lung disease			x	x																
Cryptococcosis		x					x				x		x				x			
Cushing's syndrome																				
Deafness																				
Diabetes mellitus							x		x	x				x						
Epilepsy	x				x		x													
Fibromyalgia																				
Head trauma	x						x				x	x			x			x		
Herpes encephalitis							x					x					x			
Homocystinuria		x										x					x			
Huntington's disease		x			x			x	x							x				
Hyperparathyroidism															x					
Hypertensive encephalopathy							x					x						x		
Hyperthyroidism			x															x		

| Hypoparathyroidism |
| Hypothyroidism |
| Kidney failure |
| Klinefelter's syndrome |
| Liver failure |
| Lyme disease |
| Ménière's syndrome |
| Menopause |
| Migraine |
| Mitral valve prolapse |
| Multiple sclerosis |
| Myasthenia gravis |
| Neurocutaneous disease |
| Normal pressure hydrocephalus |
| Parkinson's disease |
| Pellagra |
| Pernicious anemia |
| Pheochromocytoma |
| Pneumonia |
| Porphyria |
| Postoperative states |
| Premenstrual syndrome |
| Prion disease |
| Progressive supranuclear palsy |
| Protein energy malnutrition |
| Pulmonary thromboembolism |
| Rheumatoid arthritis |
| Sickle-cell disease |
| Sleep apnea |
| Syphilis |
| Systemic infection |
| Systemic lupus erythematosus |
| Thiamine deficiency |
| Wilson's disease |

Summary of Symptoms: Neurological II

	Sensory defect	Burning pains	Sensory hypersensitivity	Dizziness	Tinnitus	Deafness	Neuropathy	Headache	Drowsy	Snoring	Aphasia	Apraxia	Agnosia	Amnesia	Executive functioning	Paresthesias	Numbness	Neglect	Voice deep
Adrenal insufficiency			X																
AIDS								X											
Altitude sickness				X				X	X										
Amyotrophic lateral sclerosis																			
Antidiuretic excess								X											
Brain abscess								X			X								
Brain tumor				X		X		X			X	X		X					
Cancer	X														X				
Carcinoid syndrome																			
Cardiac arrythmia				X															
Cerebrovascular accident	X										X	X	X	X	X		X	X	
Chronic obstructive lung disease								X	X										
Congestive heart failure									X										
Cryptococcosis								X											
Cushing's syndrome																			
Deafness						X													
Diabetes mellitus							X												
Epilepsy									X					X					
Fibromyalgia		X																	
Head trauma				X				X	X					X					
Herpes encephalitis											X					X			
Homocystinuria																	X		
Huntington's disease																			
Hyperparathyroidism																			
Hypertensive encephalopathy				X				X	X								X		
Hyperthyroidism																			

Disease																	
Hypoparathyroidism																	×
Hypothyroidism	×	×															
Kidney failure	×					×											
Klinefelter's syndrome																	
Liver failure	×					×											
Lyme disease	×		×														
Ménière's syndrome	×	×	×	×													
Menopause					×												
Migraine	×	×	×					×									
Mitral valve prolapse			×														
Multiple sclerosis	×	.	×														
Myasthenia gravis																	
Neurocutaneous disease				×	×												
Normal pressure hydrocephalus																	
Parkinson's disease																	
Pellagra	×		×			×											
Pernicious anemia	×	×	×	×		×											
Pheochromocytoma	×	×	×			×											
Pneumonia						×											
Porphyria	×																
Postoperative states																	
Premenstrual syn.						×											
Prion disease		×				×											
Progressive supranuclear palsy																	
Protein energy malnutrition			×														
Pulmonary thromboembolism																	
Rheumatoid arthritis																	
Sickle-cell disease				×													
Sleep apnea	×			×		×										×	×
Syphilis	×	×				×										×	×
Systemic infection																	
Systemic lupus erythematosus																	
Thiamine deficiency		×			×								×			×	×
Wilson's disease																	

Summary of Symptoms: Emotional/Behavioral

	Depression	Mania	Anxiety	Panic attacks	Obsessive-compulsive	Labile emotions	Withdrawal	Catatonia *	Insomnia	Hypersomnia	Hallucinations	Delusions	Depersonalization/derealization	Déjà vu	Poor judgment	Suicidal ideas	PTSD	Flushing	Klüver-Bucy
Adrenal insufficiency	x		x				x				x	x				x			
AIDS	x	x	x				x				x	x				x			
Altitude sickness	x								x			x			x	x			
Amyotrophic lateral sclerosis				x															
Antidiuretic excess									x		x	x			x				
Brain abscess	x										x								
Brain tumor	x	x	x			x				x	x	x	x	x					
Cancer	x									x			x			x	x		
Carcinoid syndrome		x	x	x														x	
Cardiac arrythmia			x														x		
Cerebrovascular accident	x	x	x	x		x			x		x	x			x				
Chronic obstructive lung disease	x		x	x					x		x	x			x	x			
Congestive heart failure	x		x	x					x		x				x	x			
Cryptococcosis									x		x								
Cushing's syndrome	x	x	x						x		x	x				x			
Deafness			x								x	x							
Diabetes mellitus	x		x	x															
Epilepsy		x						x			x	x				x			
Fibromyalgia	x	x	x	x															
Head trauma	x	x	x						x		x	x							
Herpes encephalitis								x			x								x
Homocystinuria								x											
Huntington's disease	x	x				x													
Hyperparathyroidism	x		x			x					x	x				x			
Hypertensive encephalopathy											x	x							
Hyperthyroidism	x		x	x		x			x		x								

206

Hypoparathyroidism
Hypothyroidism
Kidney failure
Klinefelter's syndrome
Liver failure
Lyme disease
Ménière's syndrome
Menopause
Migraine
Mitral valve prolapse
Multiple sclerosis
Myasthenia gravis
Neurocutaneous disease
Normal pressure hydrocephalus
Parkinson's disease
Pellagra
Pernicious anemia
Pheochromocytoma
Pneumonia
Porphyria
Postoperative states
Premenstrual syndrome
Prion disease
Progressive supranuclear palsy
Protein energy malnutrition
Pulmonary thromboembolism
Rheumatoid arthritis
Sickle-cell disease
Sleep apnea
Syphilis
Systemic infection
Systemic lupus erythematosus
Thiamine deficiency
Wilson's disease

* Negativism, posturing, catalepsy, waxy flexibility.

Summary of Symptoms: Cognitive and Personality

	Cognitive								Personality							
	Memory impaired	Disorientation	Minor cognitive decline	Delirium	Dementia	Inattention	Slow thinking	Mental retardation	Irritability	Apathetic	Disinhibited	Jocular	Impulsive	Tenacious	Aggressive	Criminality
Adrenal insufficiency	×			×					×	×						
AIDS	×	×	×	×	×	×	×		×	×						
Altitude sickness	×	×		×					×				×			
Amyotrophic lateral sclerosis					×											
Antidiuretic excess				×												
Brain abscess	×	×				×			×							
Brain tumor	×			×	×		×			×	×		×			
Cancer							×									
Carcinoid syndrome				×												
Cardiac arrythmia																
Cerebrovascular accident	×			×	×	×							×			
Chronic obstructive lung disease				×	×	×				×	×	×				
Congestive heart failure			×							×						
Cryptococcosis		×		×	×				×							
Cushing's syndrome	×			×	×	×			×							
Deafness																
Diabetes mellitus				×												
Epilepsy								×								
Fibromyalgia	×		×											×		
Head trauma	×	×		×	×	×	×		×	×	×		×		×	
Herpes encephalitis	×					×	×									
Homocystinuria					×			×								
Huntington's disease	×				×										×	
Hyperparathyroidism	×			×	×	×	×		×	×	×					
Hypertensive encephalopathy	×	×		×	×	×	×		×	×						
Hyperthyroidism				×					×							

Condition													
Hypoparathyroidism	×					×				×			
Hypothyroidism	×	×				×	×	×		×			
Kidney failure	×		×		×	×				×			×
Klinefelter's syndrome													×
Liver failure			×		×	×				×			
Lyme disease		×											
Ménière's syndrome													
Menopause					×	×				×			
Migraine						×				×			
Mitral valve prolapse	×												
Multiple sclerosis	×	×		×									
Myasthenia gravis	×	×											
Neurocutaneous disease			×		×		×						
Normal pressure hydrocephalus	×		×									×	
Parkinson's disease			×	×									
Pellagra		×	×							×			
Pernicious anemia	×	×	×	×						×			
Pheochromocytoma			×										
Pneumonia				×									
Porphyria		×											
Postoperative states		×	×	×		×							
Premenstrual syndrome					×	×	×					×	
Prion disease	×			×	×								
Progressive supranuclear palsy				×	×			×					
Protein energy malnutrition		×					×	×					
Pulmonary thromboembolism			×	×			×						
Rheumatoid arthritis							×						
Sickle-cell disease					×								
Sleep apnea	×	×		×						×			
Syphilis	×	×								×			
Systemic infection		×		×									
Systemic lupus erythematosus	×	×	×	×	×								
Thiamine deficiency	×	×	×	×	×					×			
Wilson's disease	×			×	×					×			×

209

Appendix

ANNOTATED LIST OF SUGGESTED READINGS

General Texts

American textbook publishers have made available a number of medical texts, most of them excellent. I have listed a small handful of them here. All are written by multiple authors, and each provides a wealth of information in a package that can still be carried by a healthy adult who is in training.

Bennet JL, Plum F: *Cecil Textbook of Medicine,* 20th edition. Philadelphia: WB Saunders, 1996.—The great-grandparent of American internal medicine textbooks, published continuously since 1927.

Dale DC, Federman DD: *Scientific American Medicine.* New York: Scientific American,1997.—Loose-leaf, and so perhaps more up to date (depending on the diligence and budget of your local library).

Isslebacher KJ et al, eds.: *Harrison's Principles of Internal Medicine,* 14th edition. New York: McGraw-Hill, 1997.—This is perhaps the largest, best-distributed general text in the field, available in nine languages, including Japanese and Greek. Also available on CD-ROM.

Neurology

Joynt RJ, Griggs, RC: *Clinical Neurology,* revised. Philadelphia: Lippincott–Raven, 1996.—Four volumes for complete coverage of every topic and loose-leaf for continuous updating.

212 Appendix: Suggested Readings

Rowland LP: *Merritt's Textbook of Neurology*, 9th edition. Philadelphia: Lea & Febiger, 1995.—The excellent, enduring one-volume American text.

Mental Health References

American Psychiatric Association: *Diagnostic and Statistical Manual of Mental Disorders*, 4th edition. Washington, DC: American Psychiatric Association, 1994.—The renowned and well-regarded DSM-IV, the basis for mental health diagnosis throughout the world.

Kaplan HI, Sadock, BJ: *Comprehensive Textbook of Psychiatry*, 6th edition. Baltimore: Williams & Wilkins, 1995.—Published since 1967, a venerable, multiauthored resource.

Morrison J: *The First Interview: Revised for DSM-IV*. New York: Guilford Press, 1995.—An introduction to mental health interviewing.

Morrison J: *DSM-IV Made Easy*. New York: Guilford Press, 1995.—Explains DSM-IV using simplified criteria and over 100 case presentations.

The Net

And for those who own modems and an Internet connection, here are only a few of the Web sites that offer definitions, descriptions, new research findings, and, most important of all, in many cases, links to other Web sites.

Parkinson's and other neurological disease:

http://neuro-chief-e.mgh.harvard.edu/parkinsonsweb/Main/diagnosing/diagnosing.html

Pituitary tumors:

http://neurosurgery.mgh.harvard.edu

Other neurological disorders:

http://www.ninds.nih.gov

Kidney, urological, endocrine, hematologic, and digestive diseases and diabetes at the National Institute of Diabetes, Digestive and Kidney Diseases:

http://www.niddk.nih.gov/

Heart information:

http://sln2.fi.edu/biosci/heart.html

Dermatology: This site, the most fun I've encountered, offers hundreds of high-quality pictures of dermatological disorders. Finding just the right image is somewhat complicated by the fact that the index, as well as the entire text, is written entirely in German.

http://www.library.knaw.nl/derma-m/diagnose/dg_a.htm

Neurological information from the American Academy of Neurology:

http://www.aan.com/

Epilepsy: There is a great deal of information here on all aspects of epilepsy. Full disclosure: The sponsor is my alma mater.

http://www.neuro.wustl.edu/epilepsy/

Altitude sickness:

http://www.princeton.edu/~oa/altitude.html

Cardiology: A tour of the cardivascular system for lay people. Lots of links to subtopics.

http://www.business1.com/mdinteract/Cardiology.html

Rare diseases (The National Organization for Rare Diseases):

http://www.stepstn.com/nord

I hope these Web sites are still active by the time you need them. But a search with your browser should yield a host of fresh sites for just about any disorder you can spell.

Index

Note. Entries with **boldfaced** page numbers refer to disease descriptions. Entries with *italicized* page numbers indicate a definition. Most physical and mental symptoms are not indexed. References to them can be determined from the symptom summaries in Part III.